# Nurse Prescribing
## Principles and Practice

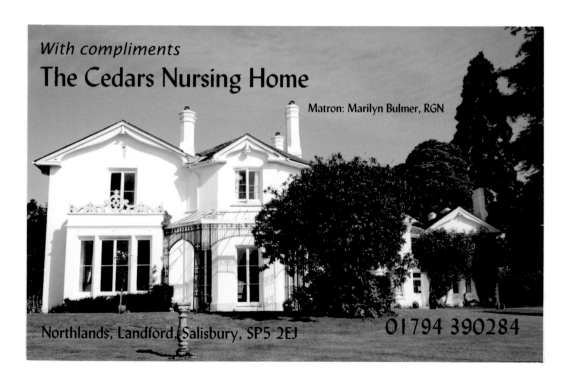

© 2000
Greenwich Medical Media
137 Euston Road
London
NW1 2AA

ISBN 1 84110 007 2

First published 1999

Reprinted 1999, 2000

Typeset by
Saxon Graphics Ltd., Derby

Printed in the UK by the Alden Group, Oxford

# Nurse Prescribing
## Principles and Practice

**Molly Courtenay**
**PhD, MSc, BSc, RGN, RNT, Cert Ed**

*Independent Consultant and Honorary Visiting Fellow*
*Department of Professional Education in Community Studies*
*The University of Reading*

**Michele Butler**
**MMedSci, BSc(Hons), RGN,**
**RNT, Cert Ed(FE)**

*Senior Lecturer in Clinical Science*
*School of Biological and Molecular Science*
*Oxford Brookes University*

# CONTENTS

# PREFACE

This book is written specifically for the nurse prescriber. However, many of the pharmaceutical products described within this text can be purchased "over-the-counter". Therefore, any nurse involved in advising the general public on common health care problems may find this text helpful.

Nurses working within the expanded role of prescriber will frequently be faced with prescribing decisions. This text provides easily accessible information upon which to base these decisions, ensuring safe and effective prescribing practices.

Each chapter examines the different groups of preparations listed in the Nurse Prescribers' Formulary. Information including product dosage, contraindications, side-effects, drug interactions and specific nursing points is presented. However, this text is perhaps unique, in that the reader is also provided with associated knowledge from the life sciences.

The authors have attempted to bring together widely available information into a single, easy to use, practice-based text. It should not be used in isolation but in conjunction with the Nurse Prescribers' Formulary, the Drug Tariff and manufacturers' product information sheets. References are not extensive, although they are supplied at relevant points throughout the text.

Readers who would like additional information can consult any of the many excellent pharmacology textbooks currently available. The authors welcome comments and constructive criticism on this first edition.

*M. Courtenay*

*M. Butler*

*1999*

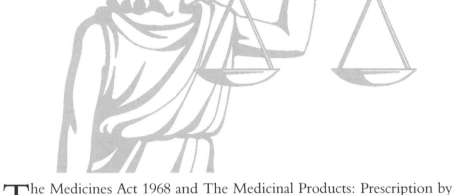

# 1

# LEGAL AND PROFESSIONAL ASPECTS OF NURSE PRESCRIBING

The Medicines Act 1968 and The Medicinal Products: Prescription by Nurses etc. Act 1992, govern the prescribing, administration and supply of Prescription Only Medicines (POMs). The regulations relating to the Medicines Act are detailed in the Medicines (products other than veterinary drugs) (prescription only) Order 1983. The Medicines Act states:

*'No person shall administer (otherwise than to himself) any such medicinal product unless he is an appropriate practitioner or a person acting in accordance with the directions of an appropriate practitioner.'*

Many nurses in both the hospital and community settings are involved in the supply and administration of POMs solely on the direction of an appropriate practitioner – a doctor. For example, practice nurses usually administer travel vaccinations, specialist nurses may be required to treat acute exacerbations of asthma, deal with convulsions, change dressings and run family planning clinics. In these instances, the UKCC (1994), require registered nurses to administer POMs according to an individual prescription or an agreed local policy or protocol.

A protocol has been defined as:

*'A specific written instruction for the supply or administration of named medicines in an identified clinical situation. It is drawn up locally by doctors, pharmacists and other appropriate professionals, and approved by the employer, advised by the relevant professional advisory committees. It applies to groups of patients or other service users who may not be individually identified before presentation of treatment' (DoH 1998).'*

The Medicines Act 1968 identifies doctors, dentists, veterinary surgeons, and veterinary practitioners as the only appropriate practitioners to administer medicines. However, primary legislation permitting nurses to prescribe was passed in 1992 (the Medicinal Products: Prescription by Nurses etc. Act 1992). This act arose as a result of reports of complicated procedures arising around prescribing in the community (DHSS 1986). Since 1994, in addition to supplying and administering POMs under protocols, a limited number of nurses have also been able to prescribe.

Provided that the nurse practitioner:

- is a first level registered nurse with a District Nurse (DN) or Health Visitor (HV) qualification or the respective recordable qualifications at specialist practice level;
- works within a primary health care setting;
- has successfully completed the nurse prescribers' programme;
- is identified by the UKCC as a nurse prescriber;
- is authorised/required by their employer to prescribe.

He/she is able to prescribe from a range of products defined in the Nurse Prescribers' Formulary (NPF).


## HISTORICAL BACKGROUND OF NURSE PRESCRIBING

The initial recommendations for nurse prescribing were made in the Cumberlege Report: Neighbourhood Nursing: A Focus for Care (DHSS, 1986). This report expressed concerns about the complicated procedures that had developed around prescribing in the community. It was claimed that DNs wasted time requesting prescriptions for such things as wound dressings and ointments from the General Practitioner (GP). The report recommended that it should be possible for community nurses to prescribe, as part of their everyday nursing practice, from a limited list of items and simple agents agreed by the DHSS.

During 1988, an advisory group was set up by the Department of Health (DoH) to examine nurse prescribing. This group made a number of recommendations involving the groups, or categories of items, which nurses might prescribe, and the circumstances under which they might be prescribed. It was recommended that:

*'Suitably qualified nurses working in the community should be able, in clearly defined circumstances, to prescribe from a limited list of items and to adjust the timing and dosage of medicines within a set protocol (Crown Report, DoH 1989).'*

A number of benefits, which would arise from nurse prescribing, were identified by the Crown Report (1989). These included:

- Improved use of both patients' and nurses' time.

- Improved patient care.

- Improved communication between team members as a result of clarification of professional responsibilities.

Patients suffering with post-operative wounds, patients with a catheter or a stoma, and homeless families not registered with a GP were identified as those most likely to benefit from nurse prescribing.

Further benefits, identified by the Touche Ross study (DoH, 1991), an empirical study undertaken prior to nurse prescribing, included weekly time-savings for nurses, patients and GPs, the time saved surmounting the cost of establishing nurse prescribing. Although unquantified, a further advantage included, for patients, a more rapid access to items and, for DNs and HVs, an anticipated increase in job satisfaction (DoH, 1991). There was also widespread support for the introduction of such a scheme.

Primary legislation permitting nurses to prescribe a limited range of drugs was passed in 1992 (Medicinal Products: Prescribing by Nurses etc. Act 1992). This was later amended in 1994.

During 1994, nurse prescribing began at a number of demonstration sites and has since been evaluated positively by patients, nurses, GPs and other health professionals. Findings have revealed that:

- Although the NPF is limited (most products can be purchased over the counter), prescribing was accompanied by initial anxiety and additional feelings of responsibility and accountability on the part of the nurse. Nurse prescribers appeared to become cautious about what they were comfortably prescribing, suggesting that they had developed an increased awareness of the complexities of the prescribing process and the importance of diagnostic skills.

- Although the training provided was found to be adequate, nurses were concerned about the lack of time available to complete the open learning package and the 2 day course. A need for more clinical and therapeutic input was also identified. Support for nurse prescribers could be provided through phased implementation, which would allow each new prescriber to have a qualified nurse prescriber as a supervisor.

- The economic evaluation of the nurse prescribing pilot scheme was not definitive. The authors suggested that the cost and volume of prescriptions has been contained, and that actual time savings and qualitative benefits have been reported (Luker *et al*, 1997).

## ACCOUNTABILITY AND NURSE PRESCRIBING

Nurses, Midwives and Health Visitors are bound by the 'Code of Professional Conduct' (UKCC, 1992). The aims of the code can be summarised as:

- The expectations that the UKCC has of its practitioners.

- A definition of their professional accountability.

- A statement of professional values.

- A means of measuring conduct (Pyne, 1992).

The 'Scope of Professional Practice' (UKCC, 1992) is a document designed to guide nurses in the development of roles sensitive to patients' needs. The scope makes it the responsibility of the nurse to have appropriate knowledge and skills for any role expansion.

The 'Scope of Professional Practice' and the 'Code of Professional Conduct' provide a clear framework for the logical development of practice. These documents aim to provide greater flexibility, and to reflect the dynamic, responsive nature of nursing, midwifery and health visiting practice (DoH, 1992). The personal responsibility and accountability of individual practitioners to protect and improve standards of care are emphasised in these documents. Within the 'Scope of Professional Practice', the need for the individual to apply knowledge to practice, and to exercise professional judgement and skills are underlined, the level of responsibility of the practitioner relating to their personal experience, education and skill. The 'Scope of Professional Practice' highlights the need for nurses to acknowledge any limitations in their competence, and 'decline any duties unless they are able to perform them in a skilled manner.'

Nurses working in the expanded role of nurse prescriber, have the authority to make prescribing decisions. Therefore, at the core of nurse prescribing is accountability.

The nurse prescriber is accountable both legally and professionally. Therefore, it is vital that they have a clear understanding of each of the products listed in the NPF and are able to provide a rationale for:

- what is prescribed;
- when over-the-counter products are recommended; and
- when a decision is made not to prescribe or recommend a product (ENB, 1998).

This knowledge must also be assessed in the context of:

- the patient's circumstances, including current medication;
- the patient's past medical history;
- the patient's current and anticipated health status;
- a thorough knowledge of the item to be prescribed – its therapeutic action, side-effects, dosage, and interaction;
- a thorough knowledge of the alternatives to prescribing; and
- frequency of use in a variety of circumstances (ENB, 1998).

A further very relevant issue for the nurse prescriber, introduced by the 'Code of Professional Conduct' and the allied 'Scope of Professional Practice', is the notion of nurse decision-making and delegation. That is, nurses are not only responsible for the care they provide but also for the care given by others, as a result of a nursing decision. In the community, someone other than the nurse (e.g. a patient, a carer or a health care assistant), will often administer items prescribed by the nurse prescriber. However, the nurse initially writing the prescription is legally responsible for ensuring that the product is used as outlined on its instructions. For example, the nurse may delegate the responsibility of applying insecticide shampoo to a mother, or delegate the application of a barrier cream to a carer.

For the above reasons, it is essential that nurses have a thorough knowledge and understanding of pharmacology in relation to each of the products in the NPF. This includes pharmacokinetics and pharmacodynamics.

Pharmacokinetics involves the changes in serum concentration of a drug in the body over time. Absorption, distribution, metabolism and excretion of the drug bring this about. The last two processes also account for elimination of the drug from the body.

Pharmacodynamics is the term used to describe what a drug does to the body, including both therapeutic and adverse effects. For nurses to develop their knowledge of these subjects, it is essential that they also have a sound understanding of related knowledge from the life sciences. This knowledge will enable the nurse to inform the patient of such issues as:

- What to expect when prescribing a product.
- How to administer the product.
- The duration of time taken to see an improvement.
- The effectiveness of the product.
- Any precautions the client should take.
- The possible likelihood of side-effects allowing the probable cause to be recognised, and a note made in the patient's records following their occurrence (ENB, 1998).

For example, in relation to pharmacodynamics (i.e. monitoring the actions of drugs and detecting their side-effects and interactions), if the nurse is prescribing oral analgesics (e.g. aspirin), they need to be aware of the possible side-effects and drug interactions of this product. Side-effects of aspirin include gastric irritation and bleeding, tinnitus, anticoagulation, hypersensitivity, liver and kidney impairment, Reyes syndrome, and fetal defects in pregnant women. Aspirin interacts with a number of drugs including anticoagulants. To fully appreciate these effects and interactions, an understanding of the action of aspirin at a cellular level is a necessary prerequisite. This knowledge will enable the nurse to identify those client groups in which aspirin should be avoided. These would include: patients with a history of gastric problems; the elderly, as this group suffer to a greater degree from this side-effect, asthmatics as they are more likely to suffer from hypersensitivity; clients with renal and liver impairment; pregnant women, breast-feeding mothers, and children under 12 years. It should also be cautioned in clients receiving a low daily dose of aspirin for the prophylaxis of cerebral vascular disease or myocardial infarction.

Similarly, an awareness of the abdominal cramping associated with stimulant laxatives would enable the nurse to warn the patient of this particularly unpleasant effect and make them aware of its possible occurrence.

To fully understand the routes of administration and absorption of drugs (pharmacokinetics), requires a knowledge of the associated life sciences. For example, when prescribing topically-administered medications to the elderly, it is vital that the nurse appreciates why the absorption rate of these medications decreases in this client group. To begin to develop an understanding of this issue, they need to be aware of the physiological changes that occur to the skin as people age, such as decreased hydration, increased keratinisation and decreased blood perfusion. To fully understand orally-administered medication, knowledge of the gastrointestinal tract is crucial. Factors that effect absorption, such as the pH of the absorption environment, the motility of the gastrointestinal tract, the presence of food or other materials such as drugs, and the general health of the gastrointestinal mucosa, can then be fully appreciated.

It is clear that if nurse prescribers are to prescribe safely and effectively and be accountable for their prescribing decisions, they must develop and maintain their knowledge of pharmacology, and the life sciences.

It is also evident from the literature concerning the study of the life sciences in nurse education that they are the cause of much anxiety for students. Their concerns focus on the relevance of the subjects to tasks performed (Akinsanya, 1982), the difficulties involved in understanding this knowledge (Courtenay, 1991), and the lack of appropriate knowledge to understand the physiological phenomena encountered in the clinical environment (Leonard and Jowett, 1990).

The information presented in this book examines the pharmacology of each of the items in the NPF. In order to help the reader understand this information, it is clearly linked with associated knowledge from the life sciences.

## References

Akinsanya, J.A. (1982). The life sciences in nurse education. PhD thesis. London: University of London.

Courtenay, M. (1991). A study of the teaching and learning of the biological sciences in nurse education. *Journal of Advanced Nursing* 16: 1110–1116.

Department of Health (1989). *Report of the Advisory Group on Nurse Prescribing* (Crown Report). London: Department of Health.

Department of Health (1991). *Nurse Prescribing Final Report: A Cost Benefit Study* (Touche Ross Report). London (unpublished): Department of Health.

Department of Health (1992). *The Extended Role of the Nurse/Scope of Professional Practice.* Letter from the CNO. London: Department of Health.

Department of Health (1998). *Review of Prescribing, Supply and Administration of Medicines* (Crown report). London: Department of Health.

Department of Health and Social Security (1986). *Neighbourhood Nursing: A Focus for Care* (Cumberlege Report). London: HMSO

English National Board for Nursing, Midwifery and Health Visiting (1998). *Nurse Prescribing Open Learning Pack.* Milton Keynes: Learning Materials Design.

Leonard, A. & Jowett, S. (1990). Charting the course: a study of the six ENB pilot schemes in pre-registration nurse education. Research Paper No. 1 from the National Evaluation of Demonstration Schemes in Pre-registration Nurse Education. National Foundation for Educational Research in England and Wales.

Luker, K.A., Austin, L., Hogg, C. (1997). *Evaluation of Nurse Prescribing: Final Report and Executive Summary.* Liverpool: University of Liverpool.

Pyne, R. (1992). 'Accountability in principle and in practice'. *British Journal of Nursing*, 1; 6: 301–305.

United Kingdom Central Council for Nursing, Midwifery, and Health Visiting (1992). *The Scope of Professional Practice.* London: UKCC.

United Kingdom Central Council for Nursing, Midwifery, and Health Visiting (1992). *Code of Professional Conduct.* London: UKCC.

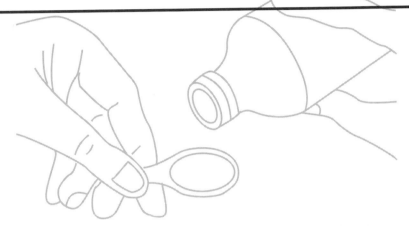

# BASIC PHARMACOLOGY

For the nurse prescriber, an appropriate knowledge and understanding of pharmacology is essential. It will influence decision-making regarding the most appropriate drug, the route of administration, the dose and frequency, potential contraindications, side-effects and interactions with other drugs.

This chapter provides fundamental information regarding pharmacokinetics and pharmacodynamics and highlights issues that should be considered when assessing clients with respect to prescribing medication.

## ROUTES OF ADMINISTRATION

Drugs may act locally or systemically. Locally implies that the effects of the drug are confined to a specific area. Systemically means that the drug has to enter the vascular and lymphatic systems for delivery to body tissues. The main route of administration to provide a local effect is topical, whilst oral or parenteral administration of drugs are the main routes to provide a systemic effect. Some topical drugs can, however, have systemic effects, especially if given in large doses, in frequent doses or over a long period of time.

## Topical administration

Topical preparations may be applied to the skin, mouth, nose, oropharynx, cornea, ear, urethra, vagina or rectum. These preparations may be administered in a variety of forms including:

- Creams
- Ointments
- Gels
- Lotions
- Aerosols
- Foams
- Plasters
- Powders
- Patches
- Suppositories
- Sprays

## Oral administration

This route of administration, which implies 'by mouth', is most commonly used. It tends to be convenient, simple and usually safe. Preparations may be in a solid form and include:

- Tablets
- Capsules
- Powders
- Granules
- Lozenges

Other preparations may be provided in a liquid form and include:

- Solutions

- Emulsions
- Suspensions
- Syrups
- Elixirs
- Tinctures

## Parenteral administration

Parenteral administration of a drug refers to the giving of a preparation by any route other than the gastrointestinal tract, by which a drug is injected or infused. This, therefore, includes intradermal, subcutaneous, intramuscular, intravenous, intrathecal and intra-articular routes. These sterile preparations are presented in ampules, vials, cartridges or large-volume containers.

## PHARMACOKINETICS

Pharmacokinetics considers the movement of drugs within the body and the way in which the body affects drugs with time. Once a drug has been administered by one of the routes previously described, it will then undergo four basic processes:

- Absorption
- Distribution
- Metabolism
- Excretion

The composition of the drug has an important influence on where the drug is absorbed, where it is distributed to, where and how effectively it is metabolised and finally how rapidly it is excreted. In addition, other factors such as the dose of drug, the client's condition, and other therapeutic and environmental issues may also have an impact on the effectiveness of these processes.

Each of these processes will now be considered in more detail.

# Drug absorption

The process of absorption brings the drug from the site of administration into the circulatory or lymphatic system. Almost all drugs, other than those administered intravenously or some that are applied topically, must be absorbed before they can have an effect on the body. The term bioavailability is used to refer to the proportion of the administered drug that has reached the circulation, and that is available to have an effect. Drugs given intravenously may be considered to be 100% bioavailable as they are administered directly into the circulation and all of the drug may potentially cause an effect. Administration by other routes means that some of the drug molecules will be lost during absorption and distribution, and thus bioavailability is reduced.

Drugs administered orally are absorbed from the gastrointestinal tract, carried via the hepatic portal vein to the liver, and then undergo some metabolism by the liver before the drug has an opportunity to work. This removal of a drug by the liver, before it has become available for use, is called the first pass effect. Some drugs, when swallowed and absorbed, will be almost totally inactivated by the first pass effect (e.g. glyceryl trinitrate). The first pass effect can, however, be avoided if the drug is given by another route. Thus, glyceryl trinitrate, when administered sublingually or transdermally, avoids first pass metabolism by the liver and is able to cause a therapeutic effect.

## *Absorption following oral administration*

For drugs given by all routes other than the intravenous route, several cell membrane barriers will have to be passed before the drug reaches the circulation. Four major transport mechanisms exist to facilitate this process.

- *Passive diffusion* is the most important and most common. If the drug is present in the gastrointestinal tract in a greater concentration that it is in the bloodstream, then a concentration gradient is said to exist. The presence of the concentration gradient will carry the drug through the cell membrane and into the circulation. The drug will be transported until the concentrations of drug are equal on either side of the cell membrane. No energy is expended during this process.

- *Facilitated diffusion* allows low lipid-soluble drugs to be transported across the cell membrane by combining with a carrier molecule. This also requires a concentration gradient and expends no energy.

- *Active transport* is only used by drugs that closely resemble natural body substances. This process works against a concentration gradient and requires a carrier molecule and energy to be expended.

- *Pinocytosis* or 'cell-drinking' is not a common method for absorbing drugs. It requires energy and involves the cell membrane invaginating and engulfing a fluid-filled vesicle or sac.

### Factors affecting drug absorption from the gastrointestinal tract

A number of factors may influence the absorption of a drug from the gut. These include:

- *Gut motility*: If motility is increased and therefore transit time is reduced, there will be less time available for absorption of a drug. Hypomotility may increase the amount of drug absorbed if contact with the gut epithelium is prolonged.

- *Gastric emptying*: If increased, this will speed up drug absorption rate. If delayed, it will slow the delivery of drug to the intestine, therefore reducing the absorption rate.

- *Surface area*: The rate of drug absorption is greatest in the small intestine due to the large surface area provided by the villi.

- *Gut pH*: The pH of the gastrointestinal tract varies along its length. The changing environmental pH may have different effects on different drugs. Optimal absorption of a drug may be dependent on a specific pH.

- *Blood flow*: The small intestine has a very good blood supply which is one reason why most absorption occurs in this part of the gut. Faster absorption rates will occur in areas where blood supply is ample.

- *Presence of food and fluid in the gastrointestinal tract*: The presence of food in the gut may selectively increase or decrease drug absorption. For example, food increases the absorption of dicoumarol, whilst tetracycline absorption is reduced by the presence of dairy foods. Fluid taken with medication will aid dissolution of the drug and enhance its passage to the small intestine.

- *Antacids*: The presence of these in the gastrointestinal tract causes a change in environmental pH. This increases absorption of basic drugs and decreases absorption of acidic ones.

- *Drug composition*: Various factors pertaining to the composition of the drug may affect the rate at which it is absorbed. For example, liquid preparations are more rapidly absorbed than solid ones, the presence of an enteric coating may slow absorption, and lipid-soluble drugs are rapidly absorbed.

### Absorption following parenteral administration

Intradermal drugs diffuse slowly from the injection site into local capillaries, and the process is a little faster with drugs administered subcutaneously. Due to the rich supply of blood to muscles, absorption following an intramuscular injection is even quicker. The degree of tissue perfusion and condition of the injection site will influence the rate of drug absorption.

### Absorption following topical administration

Drugs applied topically to the mucous membranes and skin are absorbed less than by oral and parenteral routes. Absorption is, however, increased if the skin is broken or if the area is covered with an occlusive dressing.

Rectal and sublingual absorption is usually rapid due to the vascularity of the mucosa. Absorption from instillation into the nose may lead to systemic as well as local effects, whilst inhalation into the lungs provides for extensive absorption. Minimal absorption will occur from instillation into the ears, but absorption from the eyes depends on whether a solution or ointment is administered.

## Drug distribution

This process involves the transportation of the drug to the target site of action.

During distribution, some drug molecules may be deposited at storage sites and others may be deposited and inactivated. Various factors may influence how and even if, a drug is distributed.

- *Blood flow*: Distribution may depend on tissue perfusion. Organs that are highly vascular such as the heart, liver and kidneys will rapidly acquire a drug. Levels of a drug in bone, fat, muscle and skin may take some time to rise due to reduced vascularity. The client's level of activity and local tissue temperature may also affect drug distribution to the skin and muscle.

- *Plasma protein binding*: In the circulation, a drug is bound to circulating plasma proteins or is 'free' in an un-bound state. The plasma protein usually involved in binding a drug is albumin. If a drug is bound, then it is said to be inactive and cannot have a pharmacological effect. Only the free drug molecules can cause an effect. As free molecules leave the circulation, drug molecules are released from plasma protein to re-establish a ratio between the bound and the free molecules. Binding tends to be non-specific and competitive. This means that plasma proteins will bind with many different drugs and these drugs will compete for binding sites on the plasma proteins. Displacement of one drug by another drug may have serious consequences. For example, warfarin can be displaced by tolbutamide producing a risk of haemorrhage, whilst tolbutamide can be displaced by salicylates producing a risk of hypoglycaemia.

- *Placental barrier*: The chorionic villi enclose the fetal capillaries. These are separated from the maternal capillaries by a layer of trophoblastic cells. This barrier will permit the passage of lipid-soluble, non-ionised compounds from mother to fetus but prevents entrance of those substances that are poorly lipid-soluble.

- *Blood-brain barrier*: Capillaries of the central nervous system differ from those in most other parts of the body. They lack channels between endothelial cells through which substances in the blood normally gain access to the extracellular fluid. This barrier constrains the passage of substances from the blood to the brain and cerebrospinal fluid. Lipid-soluble drugs (e.g. diazepam) will pass fairly readily into the central nervous system, where as lipid-insoluble drugs will have little or no effect.

- *Storage sites*: Fat tissue will act as a storage site for lipid-soluble drugs (e.g. anticoagulants). Drugs that have accumulated there, may remain for some time, not being released until after administration of the drugs has ceased. Calcium-containing structures such as bone and teeth can accumulate drugs that are bound to calcium (e.g. tetracycline).

## Drug metabolism

Drug metabolism or biotransformation refers to the process of modifying or altering the chemical composition of the drug. The pharmacological activity of the drug is usually removed. Metabolites (products of metabolism) are produced which are more polar and less lipid-soluble than the original drug, which ultimately promotes their excretion from the body. Most drug metabolism occurs in the liver, where hepatic enzymes catalyze various biochemical reactions. Metabolism of drugs may also occur in the kidneys, intestinal mucosa, lungs, plasma and placenta.

Metabolism proceeds in two phases:

- *Phase I*: These reactions attempt to biotransform the drug to a more polar metabolite. The most common reactions are oxidations, catalysed by mixed function oxidase enzymes. Other phase I reactions include reduction and hydrolysis reactions.

- *Phase II*: Drugs or phase I metabolites which are not sufficiently polar for excretion by the kidneys are made more hydrophilic ('water-liking') by conjugation (synthetic) reactions with endogenous compounds provided by the liver. The resulting conjugates are then readily excreted by the kidneys.

With some drugs, if given repeatedly, metabolism of the drug becomes more effective due to enzyme induction. Therefore larger and larger doses of the drug are required in order to produce the same effect. This is referred to as drug tolerance. Tolerance may also develop as a result of adaptive changes at cell receptors.

Various factors affect a client's ability to metabolise drug. These include:

- *Genetic differences*: The enzyme systems which control drug metabolism are genetically determined. Some individuals show exaggerated and prolonged responses to drugs such as propranolol which undergo extensive hepatic metabolism.

- *Age*: In the elderly, first pass metabolism may be reduced, resulting in increased bioavailability. In addition, the delayed production and elimination of active metabolites may prolong drug action. Reduced doses may, therefore, be necessary in the elderly. The enzyme systems responsible for conjugation are not fully effective in the neonate and this group of clients may be at an increased risk of toxic effects of drugs.

- *Disease processes*: Liver disease (acute or chronic) will affect metabolism if there is destruction of hepatocytes. Reduced hepatic blood flow as a result of cardiac failure or shock may also reduce the rate of metabolism of drugs.

## Drug excretion

### Kidneys

Most drugs and metabolites are excreted by the kidneys. Small drug or metabolite molecules may be transported by glomerular filtration into the tubule. This, however, only applies to free drugs and not drugs bound to plasma proteins. Active secretion of some drugs into the lumen of the nephron will also occur. This process however, requires membrane carriers and energy.

Several factors may affect the rate at which a drug is excreted by the kidneys.

These include:

- Presence of kidney disease, e.g. renal failure.
- Altered renal blood flow.
- pH of urine.
- Concentration of the drug in plasma.
- Molecular weight of the drug.

### Bile

Several drugs and metabolites are secreted by the liver into bile. These then enter the duodenum via the common bile duct, and move through the small intestine. Some drugs will be reabsorbed back into the bloodstream and return to the liver by the enterohepatic circulation (**Figure 2.1**). The drug then undergoes further metabolism or is secreted back into bile. This is referred to as enterohepatic cycling and may extend the duration of

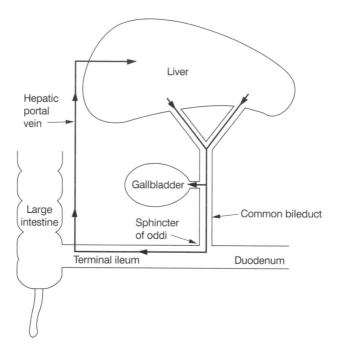

*Figure 2.1* – The enterohepatic circulation.

action of a drug. Drugs secreted into bile will ultimately pass through the large intestine and be excreted in faeces.

## Lungs

Anaesthetic gases and small amounts of alcohol undergo pulmonary excretion.

## Breast milk

Milk-producing glands are surrounded by a network of capillaries, and drugs may pass from maternal blood into the breast milk. The amounts of drug may be very small, but may affect a suckling infant who has less ability to metabolise and excrete drugs.

## Perspiration, saliva and tears

Drugs may be excreted passively via these body secretions if the drugs concerned are lipid-soluble.

The processes of drug metabolism and drug excretion will ultimately determine the drug's half-life. This is the time taken for the concentration of drug in the blood to fall by half (50%) its original value. Standard dosage intervals are based on half-life calculations. This helps in the setting up of a dosage regime that produces stable plasma drug concentrations, keeping the level of drug below toxic levels but above the minimum effective level.

There are occasions when an effective plasma level of drug must be reached quickly. This requires a dose of the drug that is larger than is normally given. This is called a loading dose. Once the required plasma level of drug has been reached, the normal recommended dose is given. This is then continued at regular intervals to maintain a stable plasma level and is called the maintenance dose.

The determination of plasma levels of a drug at frequent intervals is undertaken when clients are prescribed drugs with a narrow therapeutic index (e.g. digoxin and lithium). The therapeutic index is the ratio of the drug's toxic dose to its minimally effective dose. Monitoring plasma levels can also be used to assess a client's compliance to drug therapy.

## PHARMACODYNAMICS

Whilst pharmacokinetics considers the way in which the body affects a drug by the processes of absorption, distribution, metabolism and excretion, pharmacodynamics considers the effects of the drug on the body and the mode of drug action.

All body functions are mediated by control systems which depend on enzymes, receptors on cell surfaces, carrier molecules, and specific macromolecules (e.g. DNA). Most drugs act by interfering with these control systems at a molecular level. In order to have their effect, drugs must reach cells via the processes of absorption and distribution already described. Once at their site of action, drugs may work in a very specific manner or non-specifically. Specific mechanisms will be considered first of all.

### Interaction with receptors on the cell membrane

A receptor is usually a protein molecule found on the surface of the cell or located intracellularly in the cytoplasm. Drugs frequently interact with receptors to form a drug-receptor complex. In order for a drug to interact with a receptor, it has to have a complementary structure in the same way that a key has a structure complementary to the lock in which it fits (**Figure 2.2**). Very few drugs are truly specific to a particular receptor and some drugs will combine with more than one type of receptor. However, many drugs show selective activity on one particular receptor type.

A drug that has an affinity for a receptor, and that once bound to the receptor can cause a specific response, is called an agonist. Morphine is an opioid agonist that binds to mu receptors in the central nervous system to depress the appreciation of pain. Drugs that bind to receptors and do not cause a response are called antagonists or receptor blockers. These will reduce the likelihood of another drug or chemical binding and hence will reduce or block further drug activity. Antagonists may be competitive, in which case they compete with an agonist for receptor sites and inhibit the action of the agonist. The action of the drug depends on whether it is the agonist or antagonist that occupies the most receptors. For example, naloxone is a competitive antagonist for mu receptors and is may be used to treat opioid overdose. It will compete with morphine for mu receptors and reverse the effects of an excessive dose of morphine. A non-competitive antagonist will inactivate a receptor so that an agonist cannot have an effect.

Drug-receptor binding is reversible and the response to the drug is gradually reduced once the drug leaves the receptor site.

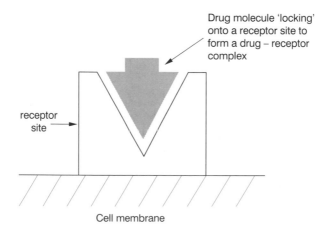

Drug molecule 'locking' onto a receptor site to form a drug – receptor complex

receptor site

Cell membrane

*Figure 2.2* – A drug-receptor complex.

### Interference with ion passage through the cell membrane

Ion channels are selective pores in the cell membrane that allow the movement of ions in and out of the cell. Some drugs will block these channels, which ultimately interferes with ion transport and causes an altered physiological response. Drugs working in this way include nifedipine, verapamil, and lignocaine.

### Enzyme inhibition or stimulation

Enzymes are proteins and biological catalysts which speed up the rate of chemical reactions. Some drugs interact with enzymes in a manner similar to the drug-receptor complex mechanism already described. Drugs often resemble a natural substrate and compete with the natural substrate for the enzyme. Drugs interacting with enzymes include aspirin, methotrexate and angiotensin-converting enzyme (ACE) inhibitors such as enalapril.

### Incorporation into macromolecules

Some drugs may be taken up by a larger molecule and will interfere with the normal function of that molecule. For example, when the anticancer drug 5-fluorouracil is incorporated into messenger RNA, taking the place of the molecule uracil, transcription is affected.

### Interference with metabolic processes of microorganisms

Some drugs interfere with metabolic processes that are very specific or unique to microorganisms and thus kill or inhibit activity of the microorganism. Penicillin disrupts bacterial cell wall formation whilst trimethroprim inhibits bacterial folic acid synthesis.

Non-specific mechanisms involve:

- *Chemical alteration of the cellular environment*: Drugs may not alter specific cell function, but because they alter the chemical environment around the cell, cellular responses or changes occur. Drugs which have this effect include osmotic diuretics (e.g. mannitol), osmotic laxatives (e.g. lactulose) and antacids (e.g. magnesium hydroxide).

- *Physical alteration of the cellular environment*: Drugs may not alter specific cell function, but because they alter the physical as opposed to the chemical environment around the cell, cellular responses or changes occur. Drugs which have this effect would include docusate sodium which lowers faecal surface tension and many of the barrier preparations available, which protect the skin.

## Undesirable responses to drug therapy

Most drugs are not entirely free of unwanted effects. However, drugs which are frequently prescribed, are highly potent, or that have a narrow therapeutic index, are likely to increase the risk of unwanted effects.

Terms used to describe undesirable responses to drugs include:

- *Adverse reaction*: This refers to any undesirable drug effect.

- *Side-effect*: This is used interchangeably with the term adverse reaction. It refers to unwanted but predictable responses to a drug.

- *Toxic effect*: This usually occurs when too much drug has accumulated in the client. It may be due to an acute high dose of a drug, chronic build-up over time or increased sensitivity to the standard dose of a drug.

- *Drug allergy (hypersensitivity)*: The body sees the drug as an antigen and an immune response is established against the drug. This response may be immediate or delayed.

## Factors affecting a client's response to a drug

Many factors will determine an individual's clinical response to a drug. Some of these have already been identified but additional factors will also be considered here. The nurse prescriber should be fully aware of these factors and they should be incorporated into the client assessment before decisions are made about which drug to prescribe. In addition, they should be considered when monitoring drugs that are already being used by the client, whether the drugs are prescribed or obtained 'over-the-counter'.

- *Age*: The very young and the elderly particularly have problems related to their ability to metabolise and excrete drugs. Neonatal hepatic enzyme systems are not fully effective, so drug metabolism will be reduced and there is an increased risk of toxicity. In the elderly, delayed metabolism by the liver and a decline in renal function results in delayed excretion by the kidneys and drug action may be prolonged. Complicated drug regimes may be difficult for the elderly to follow which may mean that inadequate or excessive doses of drugs are consumed.

- *Body weight*: The size of an individual will affect the amount of a drug that is distributed and available to act. The larger the individual, the larger the area for drug distribution. Lipid-soluble drugs may be sequestered in fat stores and not available for use. This is the reason that some drugs are given according to the client's body weight, i.e. x milligrams of drug per kilogram of body weight. All clients should have their weight recorded and this should be reassessed regularly if the client is receiving long-term drug treatment.

- *Pregnancy and lactation*: Lipid-soluble, unionised drugs in the free state will cross the placenta (e.g. opiates, warfarin). Some may be teratogenic and cause fetal malformation. Drugs can also be transferred to the suckling infant via breast milk and have adverse effects on the child (e.g. sedatives, anticonvulsants and caffeine). A full drug history should be obtained pre-conception where possible or as soon as pregnancy has been diagnosed. Women must be educated not to take medication without consulting a physician, pharmacist, midwife or nurse.

- *Nutritional status*: Clients who are malnourished may have altered drug distribution and metabolism. Inadequate dietary protein may affect enzyme activity and slow the metabolism of drugs. A reduction in plasma protein levels may mean that more free drug is available for activity. A loss of body fat stores will mean less sequestering of the drug in fat and more drug available for activity. Normal doses in the severely malnourished may lead to toxicity. Nutritional assessment of clients is, therefore, essential and malnutrition should be managed accordingly.

- *Food-drug interactions*: The presence of food may enhance or inhibit the absorption of a drug. For example, orange juice (vitamin C) will enhance the absorption of iron sulphate, but dairy produce reduces the absorption of tetracycline. Monoamine oxidase inhibitors must not be taken with foods rich in tyramine, such as cheese, meat, yeast extracts, some types of alcoholic drinks and other products, due to toxic effects occuring, such as a sudden hypertensive crisis. Nurses should have some knowledge of common food-drug interactions and drug administration may need timing in relation to mealtimes.

- *Disease processes*: Altered functioning of many body systems will affect a client's reponse to a drug. Only a few examples are therefore given.

    - Changes in gut motility and therefore transit time may affect absorption rates; for example, with diarrhoea and vomiting, absorption is reduced.

    - Loss of absorptive surface in the small intestine, as occurs in Crohn's disease, will affect absorption.

    - Hepatic disease (e.g. hepatitis, cirrhosis and liver failure) will reduce metabolism of drugs and lead to a gradual accumulation of drugs and risk of toxicity.

    - Renal disease (e.g. acute and chronic renal failure) will reduce excretion of drugs and drugs may accumulate.

    - Circulatory diseases (e.g. heart failure and peripheral vascular disease) will reduce distribution and transport of drugs.

- *Mental and emotional factors*: Many factors may affect a client's ability to comply with their drug regime. These include confusion, amnesia, identified mental illness, stress, bereavement and many others. These types of problems may lead to inadequate or excessive use of medication resulting in unsuccessful treatment or serious adverse effects. The nurse must consider these issues in the client assessment.

- *Genetic and ethnic factors*: Enzyme systems controlling drug metabolism are genetically determined and therefore, genetic variation leads to differences in clients' abilities to metabolise drugs. For example, some individuals possess an atypical form of the enzyme pseudocholinesterase. When these individuals are given the muscle relaxant suxamethonium, prolonged paralysis occurs and recovery from the drug takes longer. Different races of people are also known to dispose of drugs at different rates.

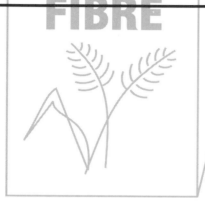

# 3

# LAXATIVES AND RECTAL PREPARATIONS

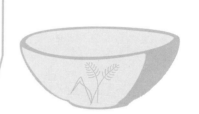

In almost all instances, the nurse will prescribe laxatives and rectal preparations in order to relieve client constipation. Laxatives may also be prescribed to aid the expulsion of parasites after anthelmintic treatment (see **Chapter 6**). This chapter will provide the nurse prescriber with knowledge to understand the primary (non-pharmacological) and secondary (pharmacological) management of constipation with particular emphasis on effective and safe prescribing of laxatives and rectal preparations.

## THE LARGE INTESTINE

### Anatomy

The large intestine or large bowel (**Figure 3.1**) is approximately 1.5 m long and 7.5 cm wide in the adult and consists of three main parts: the caecum, colon and rectum. The caecum receives approximately 500 ml of food material or chyme each day from the ileum via the ileo-caecal valve. The caecum is a blind-ending pouch from which the vermiform appendix proj-

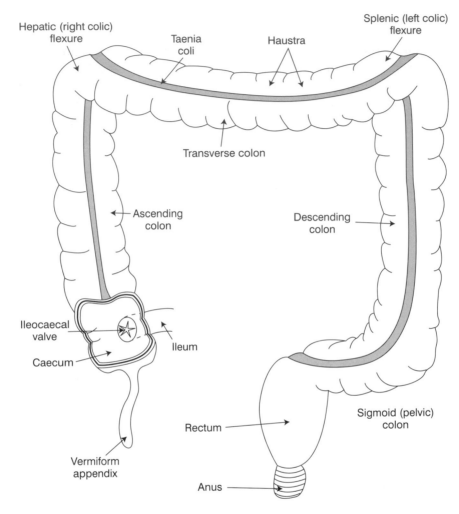

*Figure 3.1* – Anatomy of the large intestine.

ects. The appendix serves no specific function in humans, whilst the cae-cum collects and stores chyme, before it is moved on into the ascending colon. The ascending colon passes up the right side of the abdomen towards the liver, where it turns at the hepatic flexure or right colic flexure, to become the transverse colon. At the splenic or left colic flexure, the colon turns down the left side of the abdomen as the descending colon. At the iliac fossa the colon then curves at the sigmoid flexure as the sigmoid or pelvic colon. This then becomes the rectum from which the anus forms the exit from the large intestine.

# Structure

The wall of the large intestine generally has the same structure as the other organs of the digestive tract (**Figure 3.2**). However, the mucosa is not folded to form villi, as in the small intestine, and has a smooth absorptive surface composed mainly of columnar epithelial cells and mucus-secreting goblet cells. The muscularis externa or muscle layer does have an inner circular layer but lacks a continuous layer of longitudinal smooth muscle, unlike the rest of the tract. The muscles are organised into three flat bands called taeniae coli. Because the taeniae coli are not as long as the colon itself, the wall of the intestine becomes puckered, forming pouches called haustra.

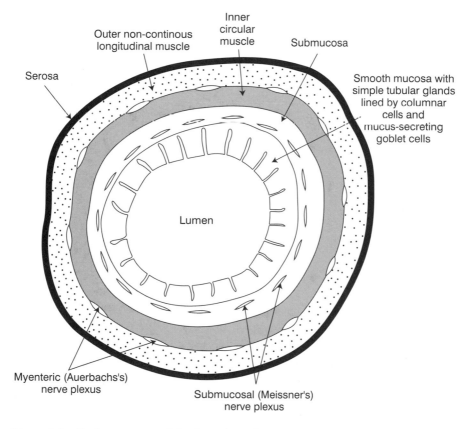

*Figure 3.2* – Basic structure of the large intestine.

# Functions

## *Absorption of water and salt*

Sodium is actively absorbed from the ascending and transverse colon and both chloride and water follow passively. Approximately 350 ml of water will be reabsorbed from the initial 500 ml of chyme entering the colon. This leaves 150 g of faecal material to be eliminated, consisting of 100 g of water and 50 g of solids (undigested cellulose, bilirubin, bacteria and a small amount of salt). The amount of water reabsorbed from the colon will depend on the length of time the food residue remains.

## *Mucus secretion*

An alkaline mucus solution is secreted which contains bicarbonate and maintains the colonic pH at 7.5-8.0. The bicarbonate protects the mucosa by neutralising acids produced by bacterial fermentation. The mucus lubricates the faeces to facilitate their passage through the intestine.

## *Movement and storage of faeces*

For the majority of the time, peristaltic movements of the large intestine tend to be slow, and non-propulsive, therefore aiding absorption and storage functions. Haustral contractions, which occur at intervals of approximately 30 minutes shuffle the contents back and forth along the large intestine. These contractions are largely controlled by local reflexes involving the intrinsic nerve plexuses (submucosal plexus and myenteric plexus) (**Figure 3.2**). However, three to four times a day, large contractions called mass movements occur, which drive the colonic contents forward into the distal part of the large intestine, for storage in the rectum. Mass movements arise because of the gastro-colic reflex. Food entering the stomach at mealtimes causes release of the hormone gastrin, which enhances colonic motility, together with extrinsic autonomic nervous system activity.

## *Defaecation*

Distention of the rectum as a result of mass movements stimulates stretch receptors in the rectal wall and initiates the defaecation reflex. This causes a strong urge to defaecate, sometimes referred to as the "call to stool". Relaxation of the smooth muscle of the internal anal sphincter and relaxation of the skeletal muscle of the external anal sphincter will permit defaecation. There is voluntary control over the skeletal muscle of the external sphincter and should the circumstances for defaecation not be satisfactory, an individual can prevent defaecation despite the defaecation reflex. The urge to defaecate will then subside following relaxation of the rectal wall.

## Bacterial activity

Many species of bacteria colonize the large intestine and form a symbiotic relationship with man where each derives some benefit from the other. However, these natural bowel flora or commensals may become pathogenic if they are introduced into another part of the body. These bacteria synthesize vitamins K and $B_{12}$ in small amounts and ferment some food residues to produce gas or flatus. Bacteria, both alive and dead, may make up as much as fifty percent of the dry weight of faeces.

Under normal cirumstances, the functions of the large intestine previously described, will enable the continued production, temporary storage and successful elimination of semi-solid faeces. This contributes to the maintenance of internal homeostasis and general feelings of well being for the individual. Disruption of these processes can cause constipation.

# Constipation

Constipation refers to the difficult passage of stools. This may be due to an abnormality of stool bulk, hardness, or frequency, causing them to be difficult to expel. The reasons for constipation are multifaceted but focus on the following issues:

## The volume of faecal material

If an individual's diet is rich in fibre, the volume of faecal material is great, and stools are large and bulky. These large bulky stools stimulate peristalsis in the colon, and faeces are propelled into the rectum innervating the neuromuscular responses of defaecation. Correspondingly, diets that are inadequate in fibre give rise to smaller, less bulky stools, which can predispose to constipation.

## Transit time

Transit time is the time taken for stools to travel through the colon and is dependent upon the muscular activity of the colon. It can be affected by certain disorders and medications. Stools that have an increased transit time (i.e. travel slowly through the colon) allow a greater reabsorption of water. This, in turn, results in a smaller volume of faecal material, which further increases transit time. This smaller volume of faecal material can give rise to constipation.

### Anatomical integrity

A mass in the lumen of the colon may completely or partially obstruct the passage of stools. In complete obstruction there will be an absence of faeces. If the lumen is partially obstructed, transit time will be increased and the characteristics of the stools may be altered. Disorders affecting anatomical integrity are curable but also life threatening. Therefore, it is essential that these disorders be detected.

### Defaecation

To defaecate, the rectum must initially become filled with faeces and stimulate sensory receptors in the walls of the rectum and anal canal. Disruption of the process of defaecation at any stage can result in constipation. For example, multiple sclerosis or spinal cord injury will disrupt the sensation of a distended rectum.

## Nursing Assessment

To be able to accurately identify the presence and cause of constipation, an accurate assessment of the client is essential. This assessment should cover the following areas:

### History

A critical aspect of assessment is the history of the constipation. Has the client had problems with constipation for several years, or are the changes in bowel pattern recent? Carcinoma of the colon, if detected at an early stage, is curable and may only present with altered bowel habits. Therefore, it is important that recent changes are identified. Other reasons for constipation may be a change in fluid intake, poor posture or a reduction in exercise levels. A change in routine bowel pattern and postponement of the urge to defecate will also perpetuate constipation.

## Accompanying symptoms

Symptoms accompanying constipation, and when these symptoms began, need to be identified. Increased bowel sounds, abdominal distention and pain may be a sign of a structural lesion. Pencil shaped thinner stools could indicate a lower lesion in the descending colon. An abdominal mass, weight loss, fatigue and jaundice can each be associated with colon carcinoma of an advanced stage. Non-specific discomfort can also be seen with the intermittent obstruction of a colon cancer. Stools that are black, or malaena, suggests a higher intestinal lesion. Colonic bleeding may be indicated if blood is mixed in with the stools. If stools are covered with blood, this may point to lower colonic and rectal disease, whereas blood on the toilet paper is indicative of anal fissure or haemorrhoids.

Constipation is also a frequent companion of depression. Therefore, it is important to look for lethargy, fatigue and other symptoms that may indicate that the client is depressed.

## Family and personal medical history

An important consideration is the client's medical history and the identification of any factors that may predispose to constipation. It is also important to ascertain whether there is a family history of colorectal carcinoma.

## Medication

Certain medications, for example opiates, aluminium antacids and anticholinergics can cause constipation. If the client is taking any such preparations these need to be identified. Drugs, especially laxatives, are a major cause in the development of long standing constipation. Gradually, over time, frequent use of laxatives may reduce intestinal muscle tone, and the propulsive function of the colon is impaired. The end result is an atonic, non-functioning colon.

## Physical examination

Weight loss, cachexia and malnutrition could be signs of carcinoma or depression. A tender abdomen with guarding, rigidity, rebound tenderness and absent bowel sounds, indicates an acute condition, perhaps requiring surgical consultation. If an abdominal mass is evident, this could suggest structural disease. If a rectal examination is undertaken, a full rectum suggests sensory deficit nerve damage or chronic failure to heed the urge to defecate. Absence of stool suggests a more chronic obstruction or laxative abuse.

## Primary management

Constipation can often be treated successfully with non-pharmacological methods, and this should be the first step in the management of this problem. Client education, therefore, plays a vital role in the management of constipation. An increase in the consumption of dietary fibre and daily fluid intake, where appropriate, should always be considered and implemented. The ideal quantity of fibre intake per day is 18 g (DoH, 1991). The client needs to be encouraged to eat foods such as peas, beans, brussel sprouts, wholemeal bread, wholemeal pasta, bran breakfast cereals and muesli. These foods all contain more than 4 g of fibre per portion, which will help to provide a fibre- rich diet. Following an increased fibre intake, individuals may experience bloating or flatulence, and it is important to stress that this will usually resolve in a week or so. If clients are not keen to change their eating habits, bran in an unprocessed form will also help to increase fibre intake. Unless contraindicated, due to the presence of other pathology, it is important that at least 2.0-2.5 litres of fluid are taken each day and that exercise is undertaken. It is also essential that clients are encouraged to respond to the defaecation reflex. Ignoring the reflex means that further water will be reabsorbed from the colonic lumen making stools difficult to pass. Encouragement should therefore be given to use the toilet shortly after mealtimes.

## Secondary management

Clients that do not respond to primary measures to alleviate their constipation or who are already in discomfort because of it are likely to require drug therapy in the form of a laxative or rectal preparation. Laxatives are medicines that promote a bowel action and have various synonyms to describe them. Those producing a mild effect are sometimes referred to as aperients whilst those producing a strong effect may be called a purgative or cathartic. Rectal preparations refer to medicines in the form of a suppository or enema.

All laxative and rectal preparations available to the nurse prescriber are listed in **Table 3.1**. These products are usually classified according to their mode of action and will be examined in the following section.

**Table 3.1** – *Laxatives and rectal preparations available to the nurse prescriber.*

| Group of laxatives | Generic name |
| --- | --- |
| Bulk-forming | Isphagula husk granules |
| | Isphagula husk granules effervescent |
| | Isphagula husk powder |
| | Sterculia granules |
| | Sterculia and frangula granules |
| Osmotic | Lactulose solution |
| | Lactulose powder |
| | Lactitol powder |
| | Magnesium hydroxide mixture |
| | Phosphate enema |
| | Sodium citrate enemas |
| Stimulant | Senna granules |
| | Senna oral solution |
| | Senna tablets |
| | Senna and Isphagula granules |
| | Bisacodyl tablets |
| | Bisacodyl suppositories |
| | Codanthramer capsules |
| | Codanthramer capsules, strong |
| | Codanthramer oral suspension |
| | Codanthramer oral suspension, strong |
| | Codanthrusate capsules |
| | Codanthrusate oral suspension |
| | Sodium picosulphate elixir |
| | Glycerol suppositories |
| Faecal softeners | Arachis oil retention enema |
| | Docusate capsules |
| | Docusate enema |
| | Docusate oral solution |
| | Docusate oral solution, paediatric |

## Bulk-forming laxatives

- **Isphagula** (*Fybogel®*, *Regulan®*)

- **Sterculia** (*Normacol®*, *Normacol plus®*)

These are also referred to as fibre-like laxatives and they will increase the faecal bulk by directly increasing the volume of faecal material which stimulates peristalsis. They may add to faecal mass by acting as substrates for the growth of colonic bacteria. Some compounds trap water in the colon by forming a viscous gel. This leads to an increase in the weight of the faeces, softens the faeces and reduces overall transit time.

These drugs are effective in simple constipation arising from a low fibre, low fluid diet.

---

## CONTRAINDICATIONS

Intestinal obstruction, atonic colon, and faecal impaction.

## SIDE-EFFECTS

Flatulence and abdominal distention.

---

## Nursing points

*These preparations must be taken with water and additional fluid of 2.0-3.0 litres per day is essential. They should not be taken before going to bed in order to reduce the risk of obstruction. Some clients will get a reduction in appetite leading to reduced food intake and possible risk of malnutrition. Clients should be informed that these drugs may take up to 3 days to have an effect. Duration of action depends on continued administration. They may be used safely in pregnancy.*

## Osmotic laxatives and rectal preparations

- **Lactulose**
- **Lactitol**
- **Magnesium hydroxide**
- **Phosphate enema**
- **Sodium citrate enemas** (*Micolette®, Micralax®, Relaxit®*)

These products, all of which are poorly absorbed from the intestine, retain fluid in the large intestine by osmosis, or by changing the pattern of water distribution in the faeces. The retention of fluid in the lumen then causes intestinal distension and eventual peristalsis.

Lactulose is a synthetic disaccharide or sugar, which is unaffected by the disaccharidase enzyme in the small intestine, and hence it is not absorbed. Lactulose remains in the intestine and exerts its laxative effect by pulling water into the intestinal lumen. Lactulose undergoes fermentation in the colon and this produces gas and short-chain fatty acids. Ultimately, these will stimulate intestinal motility and increase the growth of bowel flora, both of which accelerate transit time and increase stool weight respectively (Spiller and Farthing, 1994).

Lactulose is used in chronic constipation whilst magnesium preparations, phosphate enemas and sodium citrate enemas provide a more prompt and complete evacuation.

## CONTRAINDICATIONS

Lactulose is contraindicated in intestinal obstruction and galactosaemia. The other products in this group should not be used if intestinal obstruction and other acute gastro-intestinal conditions are present.

## SIDE-EFFECTS

Lactulose may cause cramps, flatulence and general abdominal discomfort. The other products in this group may induce colic and gastro-intestinal irritation.

## *Nursing points*

*Lactulose is best administered with either water or fruit juice and may take 48 hours to have any effect. Magnesium hydroxide mixture should be shaken well before use and then taken with a full glass of water. The client should be informed that it will take 2-4 hours to have an effect.*

## *Stimulant laxatives and rectal preparations*

- **Senna** (*Senokot®*)
- **Bisacodyl**
- **Sodium picosulphate elixir** (*Dulcolax liquid®*)

- **Codanthramer** (*Codalax®*, *Normax®*)

- **Glycerol** (*Glycerin®* suppositories)

These products are also referred to as irritant or contact laxatives. They will increase motility of the large intestine by inducing peristaltic activity. They stimulate the intrinsic nerve plexuses to initiate large propulsive waves. Chronic use of these products may lead to 'melanosis coli' (hyperpigmentation of the colon) and irreversible damage to the nerve plexuses. Spiller (1990) suggests that stimulant laxatives used infrequently, perhaps no more than once a week, at the minimal effective dose are unlikely to cause significant harm.

Codanthramer use has been associated with a carcinogenic risk in rodents and long term exposure to this drug should be avoided. It may be suitable for treatment of constipation in the elderly or the terminally ill (Laurence and Bennett 1992). It should, however, only be prescribed in consultation with a physician.

Stimulant laxatives are particularly used to treat constipation caused by prolonged bed rest, neurologic dysfunction of the colon and constipating drugs.

## CONTRAINDICATIONS

Senna, bisacodyl and codanthramer should all be avoided in intestinal obstruction or undiagnosed abdominal pain. They should preferably be avoided in children and used with caution in pregnancy, as they may stimulate uterine activity. Milder laxatives would be more suitable.

## SIDE EFFECTS

Senna, bisacodyl and codanthramer may all cause griping and abdominal cramps. Bisacodyl suppositories may cause some local irritation to the rectum.

### Nursing points

*Senna should be taken with adequate fluid and will have its effect within 8-12 hours.*

*Bisacodyl should be taken after food and not within one hour of other drugs. It will have an effect in 10-12 hours. The effect of the suppository usually occurs in 20-60 minutes but the suppository must be in contact will the rectal mucosa for the best effect.*

*Codanthramer is best taken at bedtime and takes 6-12 hours to have an effect.*

*Glycerol suppositories should be moistened with water and inserted directly into faeces to be effective.*

### Faecal softeners and lubricants

- **Docusate sodium** (*Dioctyl®, Fletchers' Enemette®, Norgalax®*)
- **Arachis oil retention enema**

These products assist mucus in the lubrication of faeces to promote easier passage as well as softening faeces. In addition, some, such as docusate sodium, also lower the surface tension of the faecal material, which then allows fluid to penetrate and soften the stool. Docusate sodium also possesses some stimulant activity. Liquid paraffin was considered the classical lubricant and stool softener but should no longer be used due to problems which include impaired absorption of fat-soluble vitamins, potential inhalation of oil droplets causing a lipid pneumonia, anal seepage of oil and risk of carcinoma from prolonged use (Crossland, 1980).

Softeners should be used in clients that need to avoid straining during defaecation (e.g. after myocardial infarction, surgery, or in clients with hernias or ano-rectal problems).

## CONTRAINDICATIONS

Oral docusate sodium should not be prescribed in intestinal obstruction or clients with nausea, vomiting and abdominal pain. Rectal preparations should be avoided in clients with haemorrhoids and anal fissure.

## SIDE EFFECTS

Oral docusate sodium may cause nausea, anorexia, and cramp.

## Nursing points

*Better absorption occurs when oral docusate sodium is taken alone and not within an hour of other drugs. Adequate water should be consumed at the same time. A laxative effect is seen in 1-2 days.*

*The arachis oil enema is likely to be most effective if warmed and retained by the client for as long as possible.*

## Choice of laxative or rectal preparation – general principles

If the constipation appears to be simple or functional and is not likely to be secondary to underlying disease, then management should not require medical intervention.

Several preparations are available from which the nurse prescriber may select. For many clients bulk-forming drugs should be the first choice, as these mimic the natural action of food on the intestine and can be used over a longer period of time, if required. For a client in whom straining is potentially harmful or painful, faecal softeners are the agents of choice. A short course of a stimulant laxative may be of use if clients do not respond to bulk-forming drugs or appear to have more advanced constipation. Severe constipation and faecal impaction may only respond initially to the use of suppositories or enemas. Where possible, manual evacuation of the rectum should be avoided. This may be very distressing, painful and potentially dangerous for the patient. Oral laxatives are contraindicated when impaction is present but may be prescribed when the faecal mass has been removed. A bulk-forming agent daily or another laxative once or twice weekly may be necessary if the client fails to respond to dietary and other non-pharmacological measures.

An informed decision about the choice of product should be made following consideration of the client's physical and psycho-social factors. Butler (1998) identifies several points in a checklist, which may be used to assist decision-making regarding the most appropriate drug, route and dose (**Box 3.1**).

## Prescribing in children

Few paediatricians appear to be in favour of laxatives and enemas for children and regular dosing is discouraged unless specifically prescribed by a

**BOX 3.1 – CHECKLIST TO ASSIST THE NURSE PRESCRIBER IN DECIDING THE MOST APPROPRIATE TREATMENT FOR CONSTIPATION.**

- Client's age _____
- Present medical conditions _____

- Specific medical problems of the gastrointestinal system _____

- Pregnant or breastfeeding Yes/No
- Effects of advice regarding:   diet _____
                                 fluid _____
                                 exercise _____
- Self-medication already undertaken by client Yes/No
  If yes, which drug(s) and dose _____

- Evidence of long term laxative use Yes/No
- Degree of constipation: mild _____ moderate _____ severe/impacted _____
- Degree of client discomfort: mild _____ moderate _____ severe _____
- Client's preference for a specific drug and/or route _____

- When is drug required to have its effects _____

- Possible side effects of treatment _____

- Client likely to be compliant with treatment Yes/No
- Client's level of mobility _____
- Available toilet facilities and their location _____

- Client support services available (e.g. relative) _____

physician. Primary constipation should be managed by dietary adjustments and these will depend on the age of the child. In addition, plenty of fluid, exercise, a suitable toileting environment and provision of adequate time for defaecation are essential. If dietary modification fails to relieve the problem then a single glycerol suppository may provide a satisfactory response

(Nathan, 1996). Stool softeners may be given to older children but stimulant laxatives should be avoided. The nurse prescriber should consult with a physician before prescribing a laxative for a child.

## Evaluation of treatment

Successful treatment should be reinforced by client education in order to prevent recurrence. This should include information about life-style changes and not buying over-the-counter laxatives. Both repeat prescriptions from the nurse prescriber and purchases of laxatives by the client should be avoided. Both will increase the chances of laxative abuse, which ultimately may perpetuate the constipation.

Most clients requiring continued treatment will benefit from a bulk-forming laxative. Some clients will require a laxative prescription indefinitely, for example those receiving opiate medication. Unresolved constipation should be followed up by further assessment from the client's general practitioner in case of the presence of other pathology.

## References

Butler M.A. (1998). Laxatives and rectal preparations. *Nursing Times* 94 (3): 56–58.

Crossland J. (1980). *Lewis's Pharmacology* (5ᵗʰ edition). Edinburgh: Churchill Livingstone.

Department of Health (1991). *Report on Health and Social Subjects 41. Dietary Reference Values for Food Energy and Nutrients for the United Kingdom*. London: HMSO.

Laurence D.R. and Bennett P.N. (1992). *Clinical Pharmacology* (7ᵗʰ edition). Edinburgh: Churchill Livingstone.

Nathan A. (1996). Laxatives. *The Pharmaceutical Journal* 257: 52–55.

Spiller R.C. and Farthing M.J.G. (1994). *Diarrhoea and Constipation*. London: Science Press.

Spiller R.C. (1990). Management of constipation – when fibre fails. *British Medical Journal* 300: 1064–1065.

# 4

# PREPARATIONS FOR SKIN CONDITIONS

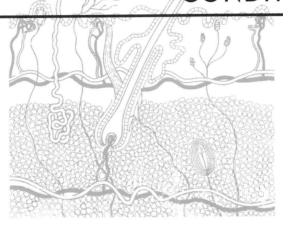

The major skin preparations listed in the NPF (see **Appendix 2**) involve the treatments for dry and damaged skin, dermatitis, eczema, and napkin rash. This chapter describes these preparations and examines their actions. In order to fully appreciate how each product works, the chapter commences with a description of the anatomy and physiology of the skin. Each of the different skin preparations in the NPF is then examined.

## THE SKIN

The skin is the largest of the body's organs. It has a vast surface area, which spans approximately two square metres and accounts for roughly 16% of an individual's total body weight.

The skin (**Figure 4.1**) is composed of two major layers of tissue; the outer epidermis, and the inner dermis. It also has a number of accessory structures including hair, nails, sweat glands, and sebaceous glands. These structures, although located in the dermis, protrude through the epidermis to the skin surface.

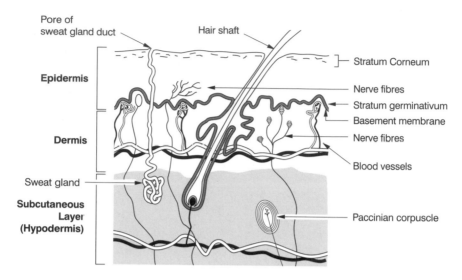

*Figure 4.1* – The structure of the skin.

The skin has a number of functions (Martini, 1998), including:

- Protection of underlying organs and tissues.

- Excretion of waste products, salts and water.

- Maintenance of normal body temperature.

- Storage of nutrients.

- Detection of stimuli such as temperature, and the relay of this information to the nervous system.

## Epidermis

The skin is persistently subjected to mechanical injury. The epidermis provides protection, and also prevents micro-organisms from entering the body. It is comprised of a number of layers. The innermost layer of the epidermis is called the stratum germinativum, and the outermost layer, the stratum corneum. The stratum germinativum is attached to a basement membrane which separates the dermis from the epidermis.

The stratum germinativum is composed of many germinative or basal cells, which divide to replace the cells shed at the epithelial surface. As these germinative cells move towards the skins surface, their structure and activity changes. Whilst still at the basal layer, they begin forming a protein called keratin. The formation of this protein is continued as they move towards the skin's surface. Eventually, as the cells reach the stratum corneum, approximately 15-30 days later, they are like flattened bags of protein, and their intracellular organelles have disappeared.

Before they are lost from the stratum corneum, these cells remain in this layer for a further 2 weeks. This provides the underlying tissue with a protective barrier of cells, which although dead, are exceedingly durable. The stratum corneum is the major barrier to the loss of water from the body. It has two actions, which restrain the movement of water, and limit the loss of water from the skin's surface. Firstly, the matrix in which the cells of the stratum corneum are embedded is rich in lipid. This substance is almost impenetrable to water and it is therefore extremely difficult for water molecules to move out of the epidermal cell. Secondly, protein inside the epidermal cells attracts and holds on to water molecules. As a consequence of these actions, the surface of the skin is normally dry, with very little water lost and it is, therefore, unsuitable for the growth of many micro-organisms. Although water-resistant, the stratum corneum is not waterproof. Interstitial fluid gradually penetrates this layer of tissue to be evaporated from the surface into the surrounding air. Approximately 500 ml is lost from the body each day in this way.

## Dermis

The dermis is comprised of a network of two types of protein. These proteins are collagen and elastin. Collagen fibres provide strength to the skin: elastin gives the skin its flexibility. The dermis also contains a network of blood vessels, and a number of other structures. These include:

- *sweat glands* which are found all over the skin, and secrete a dilute salt solution onto the skin's surface;

- *sebaceous glands*, which are found everywhere in the body except non-hairy areas, and secrete sebum which contains a mixture of lipids;

- *sensory receptors*; and

- *defence cells*.

There are variations in the structure of the skin in relation to age, environment, and ethnic origin. The skin also varies between different parts of the body. For example, non-hairy (glabrous) skin, found on the palms of hands and soles of feet, has an extremely thick epidermis and numerous sensory receptors. In contrast, skin with hair follicles (e.g. the hairy skin of the scalp) has a thin epidermis and many sebaceous glands.

### Dry skin

Dry skin arises as a consequence of inadequate moisture content in the stratum corneum. The normal water content of this layer of tissue is between 10-20%. When the water content falls below 10%, the symptoms of dry skin appear (Nathan, 1997). Dry skin can occur as a result of a number of mechanisms, including:

- *Ageing*: As an individual grows older, the epidermis begins to thin and loses its ability to retain moisture. The skin therefore becomes dryer.

- *Over exposure to the sun.*

- *Exposure to cold weather.*

- *Inflammatory skin conditions*: Conditions such as dermatitis and eczema are associated with dry skin.

Individuals suffering from dry skin may experience a number of symptoms including:

- loss of flexibility;

- roughness;

- hyperkeratosis (thickening of the outer layer of the skin);

- inflammation; and

- pruritus.

## EMOLLIENTS

Emollients soothe, smooth and hydrate the skin and are used in the treatment of dry skin conditions. However, the effects of emollient preparations are short-lived, and they need to be applied frequently even after improvement occurs. Emollients are useful in dry eczematous disorders and to a lesser extent in psoriasis.

Emollient preparations are available in a variety of presentations. Each of these preparations varies with regard to the water and oil content of the mixture. Preparations with a high water content produce a greater cooling effect on the skin, and so are very effective for individuals suffering from pruritus. Individuals with very severe dry skin may benefit from an emollient with higher oil content. The high oil content produces a greater sealing effect on the skin, and thus prevents water evaporation to a greater extent.

# Emollient preparations

## Creams

Creams are oil-in-water emulsions. Their action takes place in two stages (Nathan, 1997). Firstly, following the initial application of the preparation, water is lost from the mixture by both evaporation and absorption into the skin. Water evaporation has the effect of cooling the skin and alleviating pruritus. Secondly, the water loss from the mixture, combined with the mechanical stress of applying the preparation, causes the emulsion to crack. This cracking releases the oil phase. During this phase, oil is released onto the surface of the skin, sealing it, and preventing any further water from evaporating from the skin's surface.

Creams are generally well absorbed into the skin, are less greasy than ointments, and easier to apply. They therefore tend to be more cosmetically acceptable. Creams are a popular method for the treatment of minor dry skin conditions. *Aqueous Cream* is an example of a cream preparation. A number of proprietary emollient creams are available in the NPF and include *Alcoderm*® cream and *Diprobase*® cream (see NPF for further details).

## Ointments

Ointments are greasy preparations that do not normally contain water, and are insoluble in water. They are more occlusive than creams. Ointments are particularly effective in chronic, dry, skin lesions. Commonly used ointment bases consist of soft paraffin or a combination of soft, liquid and hard paraffin. *Emulsifying Ointment* is an example of this type of preparation. A number of proprietary emollient ointments are available in the NPF and include *Diprobase*® ointment (see NPF for further details).

## Pruritus

Pruritus may be caused by systemic disease (e.g. endocrine disease) or certain malignant diseases. It may also be caused by drug hypersensitivity as well as by skin disease. Where possible, the underlying cause should be treated. Calamine preparations can be soothing. These preparations work by the evaporation of water from the mixture, once it is applied to the skin. This has both a cooling and soothing effect on the skin. However, no really effective topical antipruritic currently exists. Emollients may be effective where pruritus is associated with dry skin.

A wide range of emollient preparations are currently available. However, there is little published evidence of the relative effectiveness of these products, and choice is often a matter of personal preference. All emollient products can be bought over the counter. However, some of these products may be very expensive, and are usually supplied on prescription.

---

### CONTRAINDICATIONS

Generally, emollients are very safe to use, the only contraindication being sensitivity to the constituents in the preparation. This effect is most notable with hydrous wool fat (lanolin) and should be suspected if an eczematous reaction occurs. Constituents in Aqueous Cream and Emulsifying Ointment include paraffins.

---

## Nursing points

*The administration of an emollient will depend on the condition of the client. It may be necessary for an individual to have a daily bath containing an emollient, and then to apply further emollients. Several emollient bath additives are available in the NPF and include* Alpha Keri® *and* Balneum® *(see NPF for further details). In other instances, individuals may only require the infrequent application of cream to an area of dry skin.*

*Individuals with atopic eczema or severe dry skin will benefit from having a bath prior to using an emollient. The bath water will hydrate the skin and therefore provide an extremely good base for the application of these preparations. The bath water must only be lukewarm (approximately 37°C). This is very important, as if it is any hotter, blood vessels will become dilated and any itching may become worse. Emulsifying Ointment can also be used as a bath additive. Approximately*

*30g of this mixture should be mixed with hot water and poured into the bath. Following bathing, the skin should be gently patted dry. If an emollient preparation is to be applied to the skin, it should be done so before the skin dries out, and immediately following the bath. Emollients can be applied as often as they are required throughout the day.*

## Barrier preparations

Barrier preparations are used to protect the skin against environmental irritants (e.g. urinary and faecal incontinence), or repeated moistening (e.g. areas around stomata, sore areas in the elderly, bedsores, and napkin rash). Barrier preparations involve a number of constituents including emollients, skin protectants, antiseptics, and water-repellent substances such as dimethicone or other silicones. These preparations provide a physical barrier between the skin and the substance causing the irritation. They also have a soothing and rehydrating effect on the skin, and help to prevent the development of infection. Zinc and Castor Oil Ointment has long been an accepted barrier preparation. This preparation is comprised of a greasy emollient and Zinc Oxide. This preparation provides a protective barrier on the skin, and the Zinc Oxide acts as an antiseptic and astringent, soothing and protecting the skin.

Other barrier preparation include Dimethicone cream, and Titanium ointment. These formulations each consists of an emollient cream base and silicone, which acts as a barrier protecting the skin against water soluble irritants. *Conotrane*® also contains benzalkonium chloride, which is an antiseptic compound. The choice of these preparations is dependent upon individual preference.

## Antifungal agents

Clotrimazole Cream 1%, Econazole cream 1%, and Miconazole cream 2% are broad-spectrum topical antifungal agent available for the treatment of fungal infections that have affected small-localised areas of skin. These infections include:

*Dermatophyte infections:*   These fungal infections are moulds that are able to digest keratin. This includes the stratum corneum of the skin, the nails and the hair. Dermatophyte infections include:

- *Tinea pedis* or athlete's foot, which appears as flaky, itchy areas of skin usually between the fourth and fifth toes. This infection is usually acquired from the floor covering of showers and swimming baths, which are lined with infected keratin debris.

- *Tinea cruris*: This infection is rare in women but common in young male adults. It presents with a scaly, erythematous rash normally affecting the inner aspects of both thighs and occasionally involving the buttocks and perineum. Tinea cruris is complicated by obesity, tight clothes, athletic supports and wet swimsuits. In the majority of cases, the client has usually got athlete's foot or a fungal infection of the toe nails (*Tinea unguium*) which has spread to the thighs on the client's hand or on a towel.

- *Tinea corporis*: This infection presents as annular lesions with an inflamed and scaly edge and central clearing. It is generally spread from the feet or the groin in adults. However, in children, it has usually been contracted from an animal, often a kitten (Graham-Brown & Burns, 1990).

- *Tinea versicolour* occurs in both children and adults. It appears as a rash on the face, head or neck.

*Candidiasis skin infections:*    These infections occur in the moist perineal area of infants and are sometimes seen as sores in the corners of the mouth of children. *Candidal vulvitis* is also a candidiasis infection that can be treated locally with clotrimazole cream 1%, but in the majority of cases, it is associated with vaginal infections which should be treated as well.

## Mode of action

Clotrimazole, Econazole and Miconazole have their effect by binding to sterols in the fungal cell membrane. This increases the permeability of the membrane and causes leakage of cell contents.

## Nursing points

*Clotrimazole Cream 1% can be used for the treatment of dermatophyte skin infections and candidiasis infections. Prior to the application of this cream, it is important that the infection is correctly diagnosed, and any necessary cultures are taken. If there is any doubt about the nature of the infection, the client should be referred to their doctor. The infected area should be examined for any open wounds as in these instances, adverse effects could occur as a result of the increased rate of absorption.*

*To evaluate the effectiveness of the treatment, the size of the affected area should be noted, along with the relief to the client brought about by treatment. Areas treated should also be observed for any reactions including stinging and blistering. Clients should be encouraged to clean and dry the infected area thoroughly prior to applying the cream with gloves. This will help to prevent the infection from spreading further. Clotrimazole should be applied 2-3 times daily continuing for 14 days after the lesions have healed.*

## References

Graham-Brown, R. & Burns, T. (1990). *Lecture Notes on Dermatology* (6th edition). Oxford: Blackwell Scientific.

Martini, F. H. (1998). *Fundamentals of Anatomy and Physiology* (4th edition). New Jersey: Prentice Hall.

Nathan, A. (1997). Products for skin problems. *The Pharmaceutical Journal.* 259: 606–610.

# 5

COOH

# ORAL ANALGESICS

OCOCH₃

Oral analgesics will be prescribed by the nurse to treat different types of pain, including muscular and rheumatic pains, headaches, and dysmenorrhoea. Some of these analgesic preparations also have antipyretic actions. They lower body temperature and hence reduce the pyrexia that may arise in colds and influenza. Depending on the circumstances (e.g. the age of the client, their medical history, or current drug therapy), one preparation may be a more suitable choice than another. The analgesics available to nurse prescribers include Aspirin and Paracetamol. This chapter will begin by giving a brief description of the physiology of pain. Aspirin and Paracetamol, their modes of action, side-effects, contraindications and drug interactions will be examined. A number of nursing points salient to each preparation are also outlined.

## THE PHYSIOLOGY OF PAIN

Pain is a sensation caused by the excitation of receptors, and the transmission of nerve impulses to the brain. The sensation can be sharp in nature and localised to the area in which the injury occurred; it may be diffuse, longer-lasting or debilitating, or it may be referred.

The characteristics and perceived location of the pain depend upon:

- The types and situation of the receptors excited.

- The pathway through which the impulses are transmitted.

- The ultimate destination of the signals within the brain. (Rutishauser, 1994)

The receptors that are responsible for the detection of pain are called nociceptors. Nociceptors are free nerve endings with a large receptive field (**Figure 5.1**). It is this large receptive field that occasionally makes it difficult to identify the exact source of a painful sensation

Nociceptors are not distributed uniformly throughout the body. For example, the small intestine can be cut and cauterised without an individual experiencing any pain. However, even slight damage to the skin can produce very severe pain. Nociceptors are abundant in the superficial portions of the skin, joint capsules, within the periostea of bones, and around the walls of blood vessels. However, there are very few of these receptors in deep tissue or visceral organs.

Several different types of nociceptors exist. These include:

- Those sensitive to extremes in temperature.

- Those sensitive to mechanical damage.

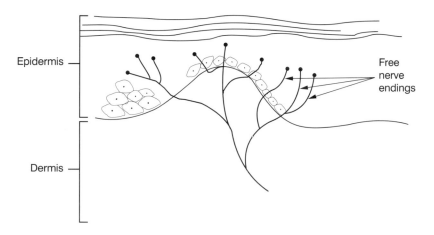

*Figure 5.1* – Nociceptor.

- Those sensitive to dissolved chemicals, such as those released by injured cells.

Stimuli that are very powerful will excite all three types of receptors. Painful sensations are therefore sometimes described in very similar terms.

When tissue damage occurs, two different types of pain can be distinguished. The sharp localised pain felt at the time of the injury and the longer-lasting discomfort felt shortly afterwards. These two different types of sensations are sometimes referred to as fast and slow pain. Their differences are due to the different types of receptors stimulated, the route travelled by the impulse, and its destination within the nervous system (Rutishauser, 1994).

During tissue injury, damage to the cell membrane occurs. The injured cell membrane releases a substance called arachidonic acid into the interstitial fluid. Within the interstitial fluid, the enzyme cyclo-oxygenase converts arachidonic acid into prostaglandin, a short-chain fatty acid (Martini, 1998).

Prostaglandins are very powerful substances, which act locally to co-ordinate cellular activity. They are effective in minute quantities and almost all tissues in the body respond to, and release, these substances (Martini, 1998). The effects of prostaglandins vary depending on their nature and where they are released. When released in response to tissue damage, they stimulate nociceptors in the surrounding area.

# Aspirin

Aspirin (acetylsalicylic acid) was first isolated from willow bark in the early part of the 19th century by Leroux. Aspirin is a non-steroidal anti-inflammatory drug (NSAID), with a duration of action of approximately 4 hours. This preparation is primarily used to treat mild and moderate pain arising from a number of causes including dysmenorrhoea and headaches. Aspirin is particularly advantageous in rheumatic and osteoarthritis conditions, where its anti-inflammatory properties are especially helpful. Its antipyretic action is also very effective in individuals suffering from colds and influenza, who have a raised body temperature.

## Dosage

Adults and children over 12 years: routine dose – 300 mg to 600 mg (1-2 tablets) every 4-6 hours for mild to moderate pain and pyrexia. **Do not exceed 2.4 g daily without seeking advice from doctor.**

## Mode of action

As outlined earlier in the chapter, prostaglandins are fatty acids which act as chemical messengers released to co-ordinate local cellular activity. Prostaglandins, formed by most cells of the body, and released in response to a number of stimuli, are major contributors to inflammation and pain. Aspirin acts by suppressing the formation of prostaglandins. Aspirin and other NSAIDs act by blocking the enzyme cyclo-oxygenase, responsible for converting arachidonic acid (a fatty acid released from cell membranes following injury), into prostaglandin (**Figure 5.2**). The analgesic action of these preparations is therefore largely local, acting peripherally in the damaged tissue, rather than centrally in the brain.

The antipyretic activity of aspirin is also explained by prostaglandin inhibition. When an individual is suffering from a fever, prostaglandins are released in the brain where they have a powerful pyrogenic effect, resetting the hypothalamus or temperature-regulating centre of the brain to a higher level. Aspirin enables this centre to be reset at the normal level (Trounce, 1994).

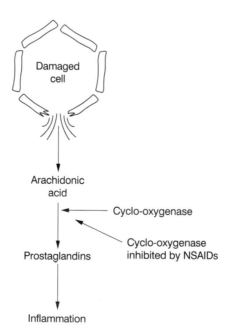

*Figure 5.2* – The action of aspirin and other NSAIDs.

## SIDE EFFECTS AND CONTRAINDICATIONS

Aspirin has a number of side effects and is contraindicated in several groups of clients. Each of these are outlined below.

*Gastric irritation and bleeding*:   Aspirin can irritate the gastric mucosal lining, causing epigastric distress, nausea and vomiting. It may also cause gastric ulceration, bleeding, exacerbation of peptic ulcer symptoms, and erosive gastritis. These symptoms are due, in part, to aspirin inhibiting the production of prostaglandins in the gastric mucosa. This leads to a reduction in the production of mucus secretion, which increases the likelihood of gastric mucosal damage. If bleeding occurs, blood loss can be as much as 10 ml to 30 ml daily and anaemia may develop if the drug is taken continuously over a long duration. The side-effects of aspirin can be reduced if it is taken with food, or in its soluble form. However, aspirin should be avoided in clients with a history of gastric problems, and also the elderly, as this group tend to suffer to a greater degree from gastric side-effects.

*Anticoagulation*:   During tissue injury, blood vessels become damaged. Within seconds, platelets arrive at the site of the injury and adhere to the damaged vessel (platelet adhesion), and also to each other (platelet aggregation), to form a platelet plug. Arachidonic acid, released from cell membranes following tissue injury, plays an important part in platelet aggregation. Aspirin intervenes in the synthesis of Thromboxane $A_2$ by inhibiting the enzyme cyclo-oxygenase, and inhibits platelet aggregation. This gives rise to an overall anticoagulation effect (Nathan, 1995). Furthermore, if aspirin is given in large doses it interferes with the body's clotting mechanism and prolongs bleeding time. It should not be prescribed for clients suffering from haemophilia.

*Hypersensitivity*:   Individuals suffering from asthma or allergic conditions are more likely to suffer from hypersensitivity to aspirin. As many as 1 in 10 patients suffering from asthma may be hypersensitive to this preparation (Nathan, 1995). Therefore, unless aspirin has been taken previously without problems, it should be avoided in asthmatics and in clients sensitive to the drug or other NSAIDs.

*Renal and hepatic disease*:   Aspirin can cause liver and kidney impairment. Therefore, patients with renal or hepatic disease should avoid aspirin.

Furthermore, as renal function decreases with age, the elderly are also less able to excrete this drug. Therefore, it is advisable to avoid the use of aspirin in this age group.

*Pregnancy*: If aspirin is taken during the third trimester of pregnancy it can give rise to a number of problems. These include: an adverse effect on the development of the foetus, prolonged pregnancy and labour, and increased bleeding before, during, and after delivery (Govoni, 1990).

*Glucose-6-phosphate-dehydrogenase (G6PD) deficiency*: Individuals with this disorder suffer from an abnormality of the enzyme G6PD, an enzyme within the red cell essential for membrane stability. The disease results in paroxysms of haemolysis that are linked to the administration of a drug, or occur after an infection or the consumption of certain foods. Aspirin is a drug implicated (Vardaxis, 1995) but is acceptable in a dose of 1 g daily in most G6PD-deficient individuals.

*Reye's syndrome*: Aspirin should not be given to children under 12 years or breast-feeding mothers, as it may cause Reye's syndrome. This syndrome is a disease of childhood in which swelling of the brain and liver inflammation occurs following a viral infection. Viruses include varicella and influenza B. Reye's syndrome is related to the virus, and appears at the time the child is recovering from the infection. However, there is evidence to suggest that it is also related to aspirin-taking during the viral infection (McCance & Heuther, 1994).

*Toxicity*: When the daily dosage of aspirin is more than 4 g, toxicity may occur. Tinnitus (ringing in the ears) is the most common effect and this may be accompanied by a degree of reversible hearing loss. Other symptoms associated with toxicity are hyperventilation, respiratory acidosis and fever.

*Drug interactions*: Aspirin interacts significantly with a number of drugs. These drugs, and the interactive effects produced, are outlined in **Table 5.1**.

## Nursing points

*Aspirin exhibits analgesic, anti-inflammatory and antipyretic properties and is used for the treatment of mild to moderate pain. Aspirin acts significantly with a number of other drugs (see Table 5.1). It also has a number of side-effects and is contraindicated in clients suffering from gastric problems, asthmatic or allergic conditions, and renal or hepatic problems. It should also be avoided in clients in their third trimester of pregnancy, breast-feeding mothers, children under 12 years, and the elderly.*

**Table 5.1** – *Drugs that interact with aspirin and the effect produced.*

| Drug Therapy | Interactive effect |
| --- | --- |
| Anticoagulants e.g. warfarin | Increased risk of bleeding due to enhanced antiplatelet effect. |
| Antacids and Adsorbents | Increased urine alkalinity. Increased excretion of aspirin. |
| Antiepileptics e.g. phenytoin and valproate | Enhancement of effect of phenytoin and valproate. |
| Corticosteroids e.g. prednisolone | Increased risk of gastrointestinal bleeding and ulceration. |
| Cytotoxics i.e. methotrexate | Reduced excretion rate and increased toxicity. |
| Diuretics | Antagonism of diuretic effect of spironolactone; reduced excretion of acetazolamide (risk of toxicity). |
| Metoclopramide | Metoclopramide enhances effect of aspirin (increased rate of absorption). |
| Mifepristone | Manufacturer recommends avoid aspirin until 8-12 days after mifepristone administration. |
| Uricosurics | Effects of probenecid and sulphinpyrazone reduced. |

N.B. Aspirin should not be given with other NSAIDs (increased side-effects).

*Aspirin is occasionally prescribed by doctors for rheumatic conditions. Nurse prescribers should not prescribe aspirin for these conditions. Aspirin may also be prescribed by the doctor in low doses (e.g. 75 mg daily) to prevent the recurrence of cerebrovascular or cardiovascular disease. Nurse prescribers should not prescribe aspirin for this condition. If clients are being treated in this manner, and taking a regular low daily dose of aspirin, they must be cautioned against taking additional aspirin as a routine analgesic.*

# Paracetamol

Paracetamol (acetominophen) is an analgesic derived from coal tar. It is an effective analgesic and antipyretic but has little anti-inflammatory activity. Paracetamol is used for the relief of mild to moderate pain, such as headaches, joint and muscle pain, and dysmenorrhoea. It is a good alternative to aspirin. By comparison, it is relatively free from side-effects, although its use is cautioned in clients with hepatic and renal impairment and individuals who suffer from alcohol dependence. It can be used in clients where aspirin has been contraindicated. Therefore, children, the elderly, and pregnant and lactating women may use paracetamol. Furthermore, it has no significant interactions with other drugs. It is also safe to use by clients receiving warfarin, although prolonged, regular use of paracetamol may sometimes enhance the anticoagulant effect.

## Dosage

The therapeutic dosage of paracetamol for adults is 0.5-1 g every 4-6 hours up to a maximum of 4 g daily. This dose is very safe. However, if this dose is exceeded it causes severe hepatotoxicity.

Child 3 months-1 year: 60-120 mg; 1-5 years: 120-250 mg; 6-12 years: 250-500 mg; doses may be repeated every 4-6 hours when necessary; max. 4 doses in 24 hours.

## Mode of action

The mechanism by which this preparation works is not fully understood. However, it is thought that paracetamol works by inhibition of cyclo-oxygenase in the central nervous system. There is also evidence to suggest that this compound acts on peripheral pain chemoreceptors (Nathan, 1995).

## Metabolism

Paracetamol is absorbed quite rapidly from the gastrointestinal tract and passes to the liver where it is metabolised. It is then transported to the body's tissues in the circulation. During liver metabolism of paracetamol, several metabolites are formed. Acetyl-benzo-quinoneimine is one of these. This is a highly reactive and toxic metabolite which is normally detoxified by conjugation (joining) with glutathione (a protein formed by the liver), which protects the liver from cell damage. During an overdose, however, this detoxification mechanism is overwhelmed. The amount of quinoneimine formed exceeds the liver's ability to provide enough glutathione. The free toxic metabolite then combines with the cells of the liver causing hepatitis and necrosis, which is often fatal. Toxic levels of paracetamol do not need to be greatly above the therapeutic levels. This makes paracetamol poisoning dangerous, as symptoms of overdose may not appear for two or more days. During this time, overdosage may be accidentally continued. Signs may include, vomiting, jaundice, abdominal tenderness, and hypoglycaemia (Govoni, 1990).

It is therefore vitally important that nurses offer suitable advice to clients if prescribing this drug. They need to ensure that clients take the correct dose of paracetamol and do not use more than one paracetamol-containing preparation at a time. It is important to encourage the client to read the labels of all medications carefully. Many over-the-counter-products for pain, sinus problems or colds contain paracetamol alone or in combination with other drugs, including caffeine or aspirin. Acetylcysteine and methionine are effective antidotes for paracetamol poisoning if given within 10-12 hours of ingestion.

## Nursing points

*Paracetamol exhibits analgesic and antipyretic properties, but has little anti-inflammatory activity. It is used for the treatment of mild to moderate pain. It has few side-effects and is safe to use in children, the elderly, pregnant and lactating women, and those receiving anticoagulation therapy.*

*The toxic level of paracetamol is not much greater than therapeutic level. Cold remedies may contain paracetamol and/or aspirin, and inadvertent overdose is possible. Clients must be warned of this and cautioned not to exceed the recommended dose.*

## References

Govoni, L.E., Hayes, J.E. (1990). *Drugs and Nursing Implications*. New York: Prentice Hall.

Martini, F.H. (1998). *Fundamentals of Anatomy and Physiology* (4th edition). USA: Prentice Hall.

McCance, K.L. & Heuther, S.E. (1994). *Pathophysiology – The Biological Basis for Disease in Adults and Children* (2nd edition). St. Louis: Mosby.

Nathan, A. (1995). Analgesics. *The Pharmaceutical Journal* Vol 255: 548–551.

Rutishauser, S. (1994). *Physiology and anatomy*. Edinburgh: Churchill Livingstone.

Trounce, J. (1994). *Clinical Pharmacology for Nurses* (14th edition). Edinburgh: Churchill Livingstone.

Vardaxis, N.J. (1995). *Pathology for the Health Sciences*. Edinburgh: Churchill Livingstone.

# 6

# ANTHELMINTICS AND INSECTICIDES

Anthelmintics are drugs used to eradicate helminthiasis or infestation by helminths (parasitic worms). In the United Kingdom, the nurse prescriber may need to prescribe treatment for threadworms. Insecticides or parasiticides are used to manage skin infestations and the nurse prescriber is most likely to have to treat clients affected by lice or scabies. In these situations the term pediculocide may be used for a drug that eradicates lice and the term scabicide for a drug that eradicates scabies.

All of these infestations constitute parasitic diseases and the human host derives no benefit from their presence. This is unlike the symbiotic relationship seen, for example, between man and colonic flora. Removal of the parasites is essential to prevent a continuous cycle of infection in the client and to prevent spread to other individuals. This chapter considers the drug treatment and management of these most common parasitic infestations. The preparations are also listed in the NPF (see **Appendix 2**).

# HELMINTH INFECTION

Helminths are multicellular parasitic worms that can be classified as nematodes (roundworms), cestodes (tapeworms) and trematodes (flatworms or flukes). Helminths may infect humans by ingestion, skin penetration or injection by insects. Their life cycles vary from simple to complex and are useful in understanding the pathophysiology and treatment of infection. The signs and symptoms of helminthiasis are specific for each helminth but reflect disturbances to specific organs or systems. Disturbances may include invasion and destruction of tissue, toxin production, obstruction, competition with the host for nutrients and hypersensitivity reactions.

Helminth infection in clients that can be treated by the nurse is due to the nematode *Enterobius vermicularis*, also known as the threadworm or pinworm. This nematode is cylindrical and elongated with tapered ends.

In the UK, it has been estimated that about 40% of children under 10 years suffer from a threadworm infestation. School children are most commonly affected, probably due to more frequent hand to mouth contact (Li Wan Po and Li Wan Po, 1992). Transmission rates are particularly high in dense populations living under conditions of poor sanitation.

Threadworms are the only commonly seen helminths in the UK. The roundworm has a much lower incidence and is more likely to have been contracted abroad. There are potentially serious consequences arising from roundworm infection, and clients should be referred to their General Practitioner if it is suspected (Nathan, 1997). Complications of a heavy roundworm infestation may include intestinal obstruction and pulmonary eosinophilia.

## Life cycle

The life cycle of the thread worm is shown in **Figure 6.1**. Infection occurs usually from contact with ova present in food or water or on bedlinen and clothing. The ova are ingested and the worms develop in the small intestine. The adult worms then migrate on into the colon. Gravid female worms move through the large bowel and then lay their eggs in the peri-anal region. The subsequent intense itching that occurs means that ova are collected under the finger nails as a result of scratching. The ova may then be returned to the mouth directly or indirectly in food. This autoinfection maintains the parasite in the host. Others may be infected by consuming food or contact-

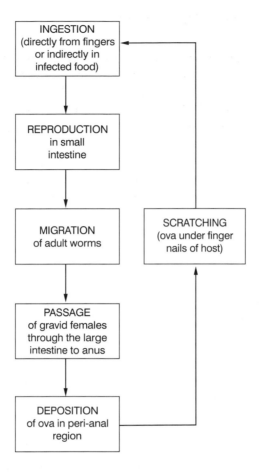

*Figure 6.1* – Life cycle of the threadworm.

ing bed clothing, bed linen or towels to which eggs have adhered. The adult worms only survive for up to 6 weeks and for the development of new worms, ova must be swallowed and exposed to the action of digestive secretions of the upper intestinal tract via the mechanisms described above.

## Clinical features

Severe pruritus ani is the usual symptom that threadworms are present. Itching is particularly common at night time and disrupts sleep. When symptoms are present, the worms which are 8-12 mm long, may be visible on the peri-anal skin or on the stools. There may be considerable discomfort and irritability in young children. Females may also present with vulvo-vaginitis and a vaginal discharge.

Diagnosis is based on the presence of these symptoms together with identification of a female worm or ova in the peri-anal region or on faeces. A swab should be obtained without washing the skin beforehand or alternatively a small piece of adhesive tape may be applied to the peri-anal skin. Either of these procedures should be undertaken in the morning on rising.

## Preparations for the treatment of threadworms

Preparations listed in the NPF for the treatment of threadworms are:

- **Mebendazole tablets** (*Ovex®*, *Vermox®*)
- **Mebendazole oral suspension** (*Vermox®* oral suspension)
- **Piperazine citrate elixir**
- **Piperazine and senna powder** (*Pripsen®* oral powder)

*Mebendazole* is considered a broad-spectrum anthelmintic. This is the drug of choice for adults and children over two years of age. The drug has its effect by interfering with the microtubule system of the worm. Glucose uptake into the worm is prevented and therefore glucose distribution throughout the worm is affected. Eventually the worm's energy stores become depleted and the worm becomes immobilised or dies. It will then be expelled from the gastrointestinal tract after several days. Mebendazole acts locally within the gastrointestinal tract and less than 10% of the drug is systemically absorbed. The remainder is excreted unchanged in faeces.

*Piperazine* tends to be the drug of second choice, when mebendazole is not a suitable option for some clients. Piperazine causes paralysis of the worm by blocking the action of the neurotransmitter acetylcholine, at the neuro-muscular junction. It may enhance the activity of a second neurotransmitter, gamma-aminobutyric acid (GABA), which also leads to paralysis. Normal peristaltic activity in the intestine then aids removal of the worm.

One form of piperazine available to the nurse prescriber contains the stimulant laxative, senna, to enhance expulsion of the worm. Piperazine is described as a vermifuge, as the worms are paralysed, then expelled alive. A vermicide however, will kill the worm, as in the case of mebendazole.

## CONTRAINDICATIONS

Mebendazole should not be used in pregnancy as it crosses the placenta and teratogenesis, or deformity in embryos, has been demonstrated in rats. It should not be prescribed for children under two years, as there is inadequate information available about its use in this age group.

Piperazine may be taken in pregnancy, but preferably under the supervision of a physician. It should be avoided in the first trimester, and in addition, lactating women should not breast feed their infant within eight hours of taking a dose of piperazine. The drug should be avoided in clients with renal disease, liver disease and epilepsy. As piperazine lowers a client's seizure threshold, it should not be used with other drugs that also do this, for example, the phenothiazines.

## SIDE-EFFECTS

Mebendazole is considered to be virtually free of side-effects with rare occurences of diarrhoea and abdominal pain.

Side-effects of piperazine include nausea, vomiting, diarrhoea, anorexia, abdominal cramps, blurred vision, rash, bronchospasm, and more rarely, drowsiness, muscular incoordination and convulsions.

## Nursing points

*In adults and children over two years, mebendazole is given as a single 100mg dose.*

*Re-infection is common and a second dose may be given after 2-3 weeks. It does not need to be given with food and the tablet form of the drug may be chewed.*

*Piperazine can be used in children under two years. It is usually given daily for 7 days, followed by a second course 7 days later.*

*Although senna is present in Pripsen®, an additional laxative may be required if the client is constipated.*

*Drug therapy is crucial if the infestation is to be successfully eradicated. However, prevention of re-infection is a major priority. Other important issues include treat-*

*ing the whole family at the same time as the client. Other individuals may be infected but are still asymptomatic at that time.*

*All individuals possibly infected, should cut their finger nails short. Hand washing and nail scrubbing is essential after using the toilet, before preparing/handling food, and before eating.*

*A bath or shower should be taken on rising in the morning. This aims to wash away any eggs that may have been laid during the night.*

*In order to prevent scratching, pants or pyjamas should be worn at night. These must be washed daily to remove and destroy eggs that may be present. Cotton mittens or gloves can be worn by children as repeated scratching is a problem. Mittens too, must be laundered daily.*

## LICE INFESTATION

### Lice

Anoplura or sucking lice are obligatory parasites of man. This means that they must exist on man in order to survive. There are three species of lice responsible for skin infestation in humans. The most common is *Pediculus humanus capitis* or the head louse. The others include *Pthirus pubis*, the pubic (crab) louse, and *Pediculus corporis*, the body louse.

### *Head lice*

It is estimated that one in ten primary school children are affected by head lice each year (Department of Health, 1996), with infection spreading easily through families.

Young children appear to acquire head lice for several reasons. Firstly, they are in close contact with their mothers who may be infested. Secondly, their heads are often close to the heads of their friends when playing. Lice will easily transfer from one child to another in this situation, with the majority of infestations occuring by direct contact (Maunder, 1983).

Alexander (1984) explains that the spread of lice is enhanced by overcrowding, poor housing, poverty, ignorance and lack of hygiene facilities but emphasises that none of these factors by themselves cause pediculosis or lice infestation. This especially applies to poor hygiene which is often considered the main cause.

Itching of the scalp is the major manifestation of the presence of head lice. The resultant scratching may cause a secondary infection or scalp eczema to occur. Enlargement of the posterior neck glands may also arise due to infection (Mead, 1996). When the head is examined, using a fine tooth comb, empty egg sacs or nits can be seen attached to the hair. They appear as white specks and are easier to spot than adult lice. Unlike dandruff, nits cannot be shaken off the hair and this may aid the nurse in distinguishing between the two.

The female head louse will lay approximately eight eggs per day, which become attached to the hair shafts, before hatching around ten days later. Maturation of the lice occurs one week after hatching, and they will live for approximately 30 days. The lice rarely hatch at a temperature below 22°C , but the rate of hatching increases dramatically with an increase in temperature (Maunder, 1977). Control of lice is, therefore, more difficult in warmer climates.

## Body lice

The body louse is seen most commonly among vagrants and therefore tends to be associated with uncleanliness. However, it does not need dirt for survival, only a fresh supply of blood. It tends to live on clothing, only visiting the skin for feeding. Eggs are laid on clothing, with the underwear being most frequently colonised (Li Wan Po, 1990). The outer garments of a heavily infested person will, however, contain active lice and viable eggs. An infestation is usually acquired by wearing infested clothing or sleeping in an infested bed.

A red rash and itching are common early signs, with the skin becoming excoriated with a pigmented eczema and secondary infection as the infestation persists. Itching is likely to be the result of acquired hypersensitivity to louse saliva. Inspection of the client's clothing will reveal the presence of nits and lice.

## Pubic lice

These lice are spread by close physical contact, usually sexual intercourse, but also much less commonly by bed sharing by mother and child, or by brothers and sisters (Alexander, 1984). The children in these cases tend to be infested on the eyelashes.

This louse has adapted to living in hair of a particular density. The head is too densely packed, however, pubic, axillary, beard and eyelash hair are perfect locations. It can even be found distributed over the limbs and trunk in a very hairy individual. The louse tends to grasp a hair on either side with its powerful claws (resembling crabs pincers), and with its mouthparts embedded in the skin. It will remain in one place for hours or days. The female will stick her eggs to the hair shaft in a similar manner to the female head louse.

Itching is the main symptom which results in scratching the area of infestation. Lice may be visible on the pubic hair or in the axillae, as may their brown-coloured eggs. Lice and nits on the eyelashes give the lashes an encrusted appearance.

## Preparations for treatment of lice

Several insecticidal preparations are available in the NPF. These are:

- **Malathion alcoholic lotions** (*Prioderm*® lotion, *Suleo-M*® lotion)
- **Malathion aqueous lotions** (*Derbac-M*® liquid, *Quellada M*® liquid)
- **Malathion shampoos** (*Prioderm*® cream shampoo, *Quellada M*® cream shampoo)
- **Permethrin cream rinse** (*Lyclear*® cream rinse)
- **Phenothrin alcoholic lotion** (*Full Marks*®)

Malathion is an organophosphate compound which inhibits the enzyme cholinesterase, in the louse. This means that the neurotransmitter substance, acetylcholine, accumulates resulting in interference of neurotransmission. Failure to transmit nerve impulses ultimately results in paralysis of the louse.

The pyrethroids, permethrin and phenothrin, are synthetic compounds. They have a similar activity to the natural compound pyrethrum, which is extracted from plants of the Chrysanthemum family. These substances are rapidly absorbed across the louse cuticle and affect the sodium channels of the axons of louse neurones. The louse eventually dies following hyperexcitability, loss of coordination and prostration. These drugs however, do not always ensure destruction of lice ova.

## Concerns regarding the use of insecticides

Carbaryl has recently had its legal status changed to a prescription-only medication (POM). It was found to cause tumour development in rats and mice that were exposed to high doses through their lifetime (Scowen, 1995). The public responded to this information with some consternation, however it must be mentioned that carbaryl has been used for the past 40 years with no evidence of tumour development in humans. Children receive only a small dose, on a few occasions, whilst the laboratory animals received much higher doses, long term. Carbaryl preparations can currently be prescribed by doctors only.

Topical application of malathion results in less absorption than with carbaryl (Maibach, 1974). However, Sadler (1997) reports on current concerns regarding malathion. A pilot study indicates that following treatment with malathion, the amount of the drug excreted in the urine, is up to ten times greater than in people with occupational exposure to the drug.

Parents who may wish to avoid using either of these substances can be instructed to use pyrethroid preparations or the wet-combing method discussed in the next section.

## Management of head lice

Head lice may be treated by two methods: the wet combing method or by using an insecticide preparation.

### Wet combing method

Some clients, or parents of clients, may initially wish to try a non-drug treatment to eradicate a head lice infestation. This involves washing the hair in the normal manner, using an ordinary shampoo. An ordinary conditioner is then applied liberally to the hair. It is then combed with a fine tooth comb whilst still wet and covered in conditioner. The hair should be combed over a white cloth or paper towel in order to see the lice as they are removed. For successful treatment, the hair should be combed for 30 minutes. This whole method of treatment needs to be repeated every three to four days over a period of two weeks (Cook, 1998). The presence of conditioner on the hair is thought to make the hair slippery and easier to detach the lice from the hair shaft. 'Bug Buster kits' are available from the charity, Community Hygiene Concern, which promotes the wet combing method.

### Treatment with insecticides

Malathion, carbaryl and the pyrethroids are all effective against head lice. In some health authorities, head lice are managed according to a local policy which rotates the use of these insecticides over a two or three year period. This attempts to reduce the risk of lice developing resistance to the preparations. These procedures of rotating insecticides are however, becoming less popular.

All three of these insecticidal groups are more effective as lotions rather than shampoos. In addition, the alcohol-based lotions are more effective than the aqueous lotions.

## CONTRAINDICATIONS

Malathion, and the pyrethroids should not be applied to broken skin or secondarily infected skin. When used, care should be taken to avoid the eyes with all preparations.

Alcoholic lotions should be avoided in clients with asthma and in small children.

All children under 6 months should be treated under the care of a physician.

Permethrin should be avoided in pregnancy and if breastfeeding.

## SIDE-EFFECTS

Malathion, and the pyrethroids may all cause skin irritation. In addition, permethrin may cause erythema, stinging, rashes and oedema.

## Nursing points

*Insecticides should not be used as prophylaxis for head lice. The wet combing method, however, may be used as a preventive measure.*

*When prescribing a preparation, always observe the contraindications and precautions. Factors to consider are: age of the client, whether pregnant or breast feeding, the presence of other skin problems, and whether suffering from asthma.*

*Manufacturer's instructions must be followed for the specific preparation prescribed. A contact time of 12 hours is recommended for most lotions and liquids. The parent or client will need instruction on where and how it should be applied, and the length of time it must remain on the body to have its maximum effect.*

*A course of treatment for head lice is usually two applications of a preparation, one week apart. The second application aims to kill any remaining lice hatching from eggs that may have survived the first application.*

*Chlorine inactivates malathion, so clients should be advised to avoid swimming pools within one week of treatment.*

*Close contacts of those infested, should be followed up and if necessary should be treated.*

*Further treatment with a different preparation will be required for those who remain symptomatic. Evidence of a secondary infection will necessitate a referral to the client's General Practitioner for possible antibiotic therapy.*

*Li Wan Po (1990) suggests that in order for nurses to avoid excessive exposure to insecticides, gloves should be worn by those nurses involved in the application of these preparations.*

## Management of pubic lice and body lice

Nurse prescribers should consult with a physician when needing to treat clients with either pubic or body lice.

## SCABIES

*Sarcoptes scabiei* is the mite resonsible for scabies, which has its highest incidence in teenagers, and children aged 8 to 12 years (Nathan, 1997). Scabies infestation is also increasing, with outbreaks in closed communities such as hospitals and nursing homes (Li Wan Po, 1990). Personal contact is normally necessary to acquire the mite, with clothing and bedding not thought to be important in the transmission of infection.

The female mite burrows through the stratum corneum of the skin and lays its eggs just above the boundary between the epidermis and dermis (see **Chapter 4** for a description of the skin). The mite normally remains there for the duration of its life, which is approximately thirty days. Two or three eggs are laid daily, which hatch after about four days. Common sites for burrows are the finger webs and wrists. However, the palms of the hands, soles of the feet, penis, scrotum, buttocks, and axillae may be involved.

An allergic response to the mite's coat, saliva and faeces is thought to be responsible for the major symptom of severe itching. Areas of itching may be widespread, with secondary skin infection and skin damage present, due to excessive scratching. Secondary infection may take the form of impetigo or pustules.

The presence of burrows aids confirmation of diagnosis, and these can be scraped to reveal the mite and eggs (Mead, 1996).

## Preparations for the treatment of scabies

These include:

- **Malathion alcoholic lotions** (*Prioderm*® lotion)
- **Malathion aqueous lotions** (*Derbac-M*® liquid, *Quellada M*® liquid)
- **Permethrin dermal cream** (*Lyclear*® dermal cream)

---

### CONTRAINDICATIONS AND SIDE-EFFECTS

See previous section on the management of head lice.

---

*Nursing points*

*As alcoholic preparations are more likely to cause irritation to excoriated skin and the genitalia, aqueous preparations are preferable.*

*They should be applied to clean, dry and cool skin, covering all body surfaces. A hot bath is not necessary and this may, indeed, increase systemic absorption and remove the drugs from their site of action. Particular attention should be paid to the finger webs and brushing lotion under the ends of the nails. The scalp, neck, face and ears do need to be treated in the very young and the elderly. These areas should also be treated in the immunocompromised and those that are experiencing treatment failure.*

*Clients should not wash their hands after application, as hands need to be treated. Re-application is essential after handwashing.*

*All members of an affected household should be treated.*

*Provided the preparation has been applied adequately, then one application is usually sufficient.*

*Once only, normal laundering is sufficient for the client's clothing and bedding. It is normal for itching to persist for two to three weeks after treatment, so itching should not be regarded as treatment failure. Calamine lotion may be applied to try and control itching. Itching that persists after three weeks may mean treatment failure and a referral to the General Practitioner should be made to confirm the diagnosis.*

*Evidence of a secondary infection also warrants a General Practitioner referral as antibiotic therapy may be required.*

# References

Alexander J. (1984). *Arthropods and Human Skin.* Berlin: Springer-Verlag.

Cook R. (1998). Treatment of head lice. *Nursing Standard* 12 (18): 49–52.

Department of Health (1996). *The Prevention and Treatment of Head Lice.* (Leaflet, March 1996 (07)). London: Department of Health.

Li Wan Po A. (1990). *Non-Prescription Drugs* (2nd edition). Oxford: Blackwell Scientific Publications.

Li Wan Po A. and Li Wan Po G. (1992). *OTC Medications: Symptoms and Treatments of Common Illnesses.* Oxford: Blackwell Scientific Publications.

Maibach H.I. (1974). Percutaneous penetration of some pesticides and herbicides in man. *Toxicology and Applied Pharmacology* 28: 126–132.

Maunder J.W. (1977). Parasites and Man. Human lice: biology and control. *Royal Society of Health Journal* 1: 29–32.

Maunder J.W. (1983). The appreciation of lice. *Proceedings of the Royal Institute of Great Britain* 55: 1–31.

Mead M. (1996). Scabies and lice. *Practice Nurse.* 20 Sept: 336–337.

Nathan A. (1997). Anthelmintics. *The Pharmaceutical Journal* 258: 770–771.

Nathan A. (1997). Treatments for scabies. *The Pharmaceutical Journal* 259: 331–332.

Sadler C. (1997). A lousy headache. *Community Nurse* 3(10): 8.

Scowen P. (1995). Government restricts the use of carbaryl for head lice. *Professional Care of Mother and Child* 5(6): 163–165.

# 7

# WOUND DRESSINGS

A variety of wound management and related products are listed in the Nurse Prescribers' Formulary (see **Appendix 2**). This chapter looks specifically at the wound dressings available to nurse prescribers. In order to appreciate the different functions of wound dressings, the chapter commences with a description of the physiology of wound healing. The different types of dressings and the role they play in wound care are then examined.

## THE PHYSIOLOGY OF WOUND HEALING

The skin protects us against a number of environmental hazards (see **Chapter 4** for a full discussion of the functions of the skin). During wounding, there is a breakdown in these protective functions. For example, micro-organisms are able to enter the deeper tissues of the body and cause infection. In burn injuries, large areas of the skin's surface may be damaged to such an extent that fluid loss may become life threatening.

Wounds can be classified by the layers of tissue involved. In superficial wounds, only the epidermis is effected. In partial thickness wounds, injury extends as far as the dermis. Wounds that involve the subcutaneous fat or deeper layers are classified as full thickness wounds.

Several causes of wounding have been identified by Dealey (1994) and described as those arising through:

- *Trauma* (i.e. mechanical, chemical, or physical).
- *Surgery.*
- *Ischaemia* (e.g. arterial leg ulcer).
- *Pressure* (e.g. pressure sore).

Incision wounds, closed by suturing, require only the formation of a small quantity of new tissue. This is called healing by primary intention and is accomplished within several days. However, in wounds caused by trauma where there is tissue loss, the formation of new tissue is essential. This new tissue fills the wound and is then covered by epithelium. This is called healing by secondary intention and can take weeks or months.

Regardless of the nature of the tissue damage, the process of healing occurs in three overlapping phases.

- Inflammation.
- Proliferation.
- Maturation.

## Inflammation

Following tissue damage, bleeding generally occurs. A network of molecules, produced by fibrinogen, bring the wound edges in loose approximation. Fibrin (an insoluble protein which forms the basic framework of a blood clot) and other proteins dry at the surface, and a scab is formed. This prevents further fluid loss and bacterial invasion. Meanwhile, serum proteins and white cells leak from blood vessels surrounding the wound. This accumulation of fluid in the tissue gives rise to the signs of inflammation (i.e. swelling, heat, redness, and pain), and occurs within minutes of the injury. Following this, neutrophils and macrophages move into the damaged tissue to remove debris and ingest bacteria.

## Proliferation

Following the inflammatory phase, tissue proliferation takes place. This phase involves:

- The formation of a network of new blood vessels in a collagen rich matrix (i.e. granulation), and the appearance of strands of collagen in the body of the wound.

- Contraction of the wound which minimises its size.

- Epithelialisation, which involves the epithelial cells on the wound surface turning down over the edge of the underlying dermis and growing under the dried scab (**Figure 7.1**).

## Maturation

During the final stage of healing, the wound becomes less vascularised, as there is less need to bring blood cells to the wound site. The wound is also strengthened by the rearrangement of collagen fibres and the scar tissue is gradually remodelled, becoming comparable to normal tissue.

## WOUND ASSESSMENT

Good wound management requires an accurate assessment, so that the best possible conditions for healing can be provided. The assessment must take into consideration the client's general condition, their environment and social circumstances, as well as the wound itself.

A wound assessment should include the following (Dunford, 1997):

- The position and size of the wound.

- The tissue type (e.g. sloughy or necrotic).

- The amount of exudate.

- The presence or absence of infection.

- The presence or absence of pain.

- The possibility of a sinus.

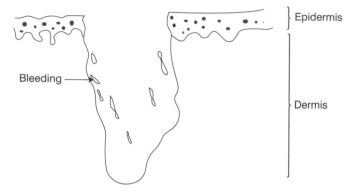

Bleeding at injury site immediately following injury

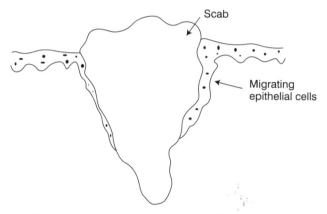

A scab has formed after several hours + epithelial cells on
wound surface are turning down over the edges of the
underlying dermis + growing under the dried scab

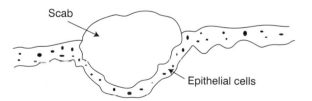

Epithelial cells have migrated and now cover the full area
beneath the scab

*Figure 7.1* – The stages in skin regeneration following injury.

Thomas (1990) has described a simple wound classification system, representing both the different types of wound, and the stages of healing through which a single wound may pass. His classification is as follows:

- *Black and necrotic* – covered with a hard, dry, black necrotic layer.

- *Yellow and sloughy* – covered (or filled) with a soft yellow slough.

- *Clean with significant tissue loss* (granulating).

- *Clean and superficial* (epithelialising).

## The function of a wound dressing

Wound dressings are available in a wide range of physical forms with a variety of differing properties. There is no single dressing suitable for all types of wounds, and often a number of dressing types will need to be used during the healing of a single wound. It is therefore important to have an understanding of the functions of each dressing type.

Dressings may perform one or more of the functions listed below:

- *The maintenance of high humidity at the wound/dressing interface.* This speeds up the epithelialisation process, reduces pain and breaks down necrotic tissue.

- *The removal of excess exudate* thus preventing the maceration of tissue.

- *Gaseous exchange*, which is thought to be of benefit during some stages of the healing process.

- *The provision of thermal insulation.* A constant temperature of 37°C promotes both macrophage and mitotic activity during granulation and epithelialisation.

- *Impermeablity to bacteria.* Preventing airborne organisms, and organisms on the surface of the skin from entering the wound.

- *Freedom from particles and toxic wound contaminants.* Older dressings such as gauze tissue or gamgee, shed particles into the wound, renewing or prolonging the inflammatory process. Modern wound management products do not cause this problem.

- *Removal without causing trauma.* Dressings that have adhered to the wound surface will, on removal, disrupt tissue and further delay healing.

(*See* Dealey, 1994 for a fuller discussion of the above points).

Prior to the selection of a dressing, it is essential to determine what the wound requires to promote healing. The requirements of the wound (e.g. promotion of debridement, granulation or epithelialisation), can then be compared with the properties of each of the available dressings.

The functions of a dressing during these various stages of healing have been identified (Thomas, 1990: see **Table 7.1**).

For wounds that require an external absorbent protective dressing, a number of absorbent cottons, lints, and gauzes are available for nurse prescribers. Primary dressings in the NPF for clean, low exudate wounds include Absorbent Perforated Plastic Film Faced Dressing (e.g. *Melolin*®).

Vapour permeable film dressings, permeable to water vapour, oxygen and other gases (but not to water or bacteria), are commonly used to isolate an area, (e.g. a pressure sore), from maceration and friction. Film dressings include, *Opsite Flexigrid*®, *Tegaderm*®, and *Bioclusive*.®

Dressings suitable for clean wounds with a medium to high exudate include Paraffin gauze dressing, and Knitted Varicose Primary Dressings. These dressings are non-adherent to the wound, have a superimposed absorbent pad, and so are effective on ulcerative and other granulating wounds.

The cells of the dermis and the deeper layers of the epidermis are normally bathed in tissue fluid. If damage to the skin occurs, these tissues dry out. A

**Table 7.1** – *The functions of a wound dressing*

| Wound Type | Dressing Function |
|---|---|
| Dry, necrotic wounds | Moisture retention |
| Slough-covered wounds | Moisture retention |
| | Fluid absorption |
| | Odour absorption* |
| | Antimicrobial properties* |
| Clean, exuding wounds | Fluid absorption |
| (granulating) | Odour absorption* |
| | Antimicrobial properties* |
| | Thermal insulation |
| Dry, low exudate | Moisture retention |
| wounds (epithelialising) | Low adherence |
| | Thermal insulation |

* Not always required

wound that is exposed to the atmosphere will normally form a scab of cellular debris and protein. However, by covering the wound with an occlusive dressing, a moist atmosphere is maintained and the formation of a scab prevented. It has been shown by Winter (1962) that crusted wounds epithelialise more slowly than a wound that has been covered.

A number of occlusive and semi-occlusive dressings are available to nurse prescribers. These include, alginates, hydrocolloids, hydrogels, and foam dressings. These products and their uses are described below.

## Hydrocolloids

Hydrocolloid dressings are made from cellulose, gelatin and pectins and have a backing of polyurethane film or foam. A number of these products are available as a paste, and others have a border ensuring greater adhesion. When placed in contact with wound exudate, these dressings absorb water and swell to form a gel. This gel forms a moist environment under the dressing and so promotes wound healing. Examples of hydrocolloids include:

- *Comfeel*®
- *Granuflex*®
- *Tegasorb*®

*Indications for use:* Hydrocolloid dressings should be used on granulating wounds, which have low to moderate exudate. This includes pressure sores, leg ulcers, surgical wounds, and minor burns. They can also be used effectively in the management of blisters, and to facilitate rehydration and autolytic debridement of dry, sloughy or necrotic wounds. The barrier properties of these products prevent the spread of micro-organisms.

### CONTRAINDICATIONS

Hydrocolloid dressings are not suitable for infected wounds. Heavy exudate leads to frequent dressing changes. These dressings should also be avoided in clients who have a sensitivity to the hydrocolloid or its constituents.

## Application of dressings

The choice of hydrocolloid will depend on the condition of the wound, and the individual environmental and social needs of the client. Hydrocolloids come in a variety of sizes, some being more absorbent than others. All hydrocolloids are impermeable to water, and therefore, can remain in place during showering or bathing. Secondary dressings are unnecessary.

Adhesion of some of these dressings can be a problem with dressing edges rolling off. This can be prevented in a number of ways (Bux, 1996):

- Choose a dressing that allows a minimum overlap of 2 cm from the margin of the wound.

- Cover the dressing with an adhesive retention sheet if the product is likely to become disturbed by movement.

- Warm the dressing between the hands to make it more pliable (whilst maintaining asepsis).

- Stop the patient mobilising or putting weight on the dressing for twenty minutes following application. This allows the adhesive to take full effect.

Ideally, these dressings should be left in place for 4-5 days. However, if an infection is present, they will need to be changed more frequently, so that the wound site can be checked. Therefore, an alternative dressing may be more appropriate.

## Hydrogels

Hydrogels are made from a co-polymer starch and are capable of retaining significant volumes of water. Examples include:

- *Intrasite Gel®*
- *Nu-Gel®*
- *Purilon Gel®*
- *Sterigel®*

Two types of Hydrogels are available:

- *Amorphous products* (e.g. *Intrasite Gel*®) have no firm structure and as moisture is absorbed their viscosity is reduced.

- *Sheet hydrogels* (e.g. *Geliperm*®) whose structure is retained as water is absorbed.

*Indications for use:*   When applied, hydrogel dressings either lose or absorb water depending on the state of hydration of the wound. These dressings are used primarily in dry "sloughy" or necrotic wounds; lightly exuding wounds; granulating wounds. These products can also be used in the treatment of malodourous, fungating wounds, acting as a carrier for metronidazole.

## CONTRAINDICATIONS

Hydrogel dressings are not suitable for infected or heavily exudating wounds. Some preparations may cause an allergic reaction. If this occurs, the treatment should be stopped. Wounds that are clinically infected with *Pseudomonas* species should not be treated with sheet hydrogels.

## Application of dressings

The needs of the client and the condition of the wound should be assessed prior to the selection of the dressing. When using amorphous products, a thick layer of gel should be applied to the surface of the wound, followed by a secondary dressing. Sheet hydrogels, once applied to the wound, also need to be covered with a secondary dressing. These should then be changed every 3-4 days. When dressings are applied to dry wounds, it is recommended that they are changed daily. In wounds with abundant exudate, perforated plastic film dressing, followed by an absorbent pad, may be used as the secondary dressing. In wounds with low levels of exudate, vapour permeable adhesive film dressings can be used.

## Foam Dressings

These dressings take the form of flat foam dressings and include:

- *Lyofoam®*
- *Allevyn®*
- *Spyrosorb®*
- *Cavi-care®* (not on the Nurse Prescribers' list)
- *Allevyn Cavity Wound Dressing®* (Not on the Nurse Prescribers' list)

Each of these dressings are very different with regards to composition, and the management of each varies greatly. However, generally, these products encourage healing by absorbing exudate and maintaining a moist environment. They are not recommended for dry superficial wounds but tend to be used on exuding, granulating wounds. A secondary dressing is not normally required.

**Lyofoam®:** *Lyofoam®* can be used on moderately exuding granulating wounds and sloughy wounds, but are unsuitable for dry wounds. *Lyofoam C®* is suitable for malodorous wounds. These products have a backing, which is adhesive and waterproof. It is important when applying these dressings that they overlap the wound edges by 2-3 cm. This is because the fluid absorbed from the wound travels sideways across the face of the dressing. *Lyofoam®* dressings should initially be changed each day but as the exudate lessens, they can be left *in situ* for 7 days.

**Allevyn®:** This product consists of polyurethane foam bonded to a vapour permeable polyurethane film. A plastic net covers the surface of the dressing to prevent it from adhering to granulating tissue. The outer layer is bacteria and waterproof. *Allevyn®* dressings should be used to treat light to moderately exuding wounds. They can be left on a clean non-infected wound for 3 to 4 days. However, if exudate is copious they will require changing more frequently.

**Spyrosorb®:** This layered polyurethane foam film dressing is an absorbent vapour permeable dressing, which can be used to dress granulating wounds with light to moderate exudate. These products should not be used on wounds that are clinically infected. Dressings require changing when wound exudate is within 1 cm of the edges of the dressing or, after they have been *in situ* for 5-7 days.

**Cavi-Care®:** This product is a soft conforming cavity wound dressing. It should be used in deep cavity wounds that are granulating, and broad excision wounds such as pilonidal sinus excision, peri-anal wounds, perineal wounds and pressure sores. *Cavi-Care®* should not be used in wounds that are clinically infected, or in deep narrow wounds. If applied to deep narrow wounds, small pieces of the foam may become left in the wound. *Cavi-Care®* consists of two separate solutions, that should be mixed thoroughly together, for 15 seconds immediately before use. The resultant foam is then poured into the wound where it expands to form a 'stent'. This 'stent' should be cleaned daily by soaking in an Aqueous Chlorhexidine solution (0.5%). It is important that it is then rinsed and gently squeezed in tap water to remove traces of the chlorhexidine, which may irritate the wound and surrounding area. *Cavi-Care®* dressings can be used for a week or longer. However, as the wound gradually decreases in size, this time interval will need to be reduced, as a smaller 'stent' will be required.

***Allevyn Cavity Wound Dressing®***: *Allevyn Cavity Wound Dressing®* is for cavity wounds that are producing exudate. It is made of foam chippings in a perforated film. A suitable sized dressing must be placed in situ in the cavity followed by a dressing retention sheet. This can then be held in place by tape.

## Alginates

Alginate dressings contain calcium alginate, which is derived from seaweed. These products, in the presence of wound exudate, change from a fibrous structure to a gel, which is believed to facilitate healing. Examples of alginates include:

- *Keltogel®*
- *Kaltostat®*
- *Sorbsan®*
- *Tegagen®*

### Indications for use

Alginate dressings are of little value if applied to dry, or lightly exuding wounds. Their primary use is in the treatment of exuding granulating wounds including leg ulcers, acute surgical wounds, sinuses and other cavity wounds (e.g. pressure sores). Malodorous wounds can also be effectively treated with the alginate *Sorbsan®*.

> **CONTRAINDICATIONS**
>
> Alginate dressings are not the dressing of choice for infected wounds. They are also unsuitable for very dry wounds or wounds covered with hard necrotic tissue. Alginates should not be used with topical antimicrobial or antibiotic agents they may prevent the gelling process from occurring.

## Application of dressings

Alginate dressings come in a variety of forms, including flat dressings, rope or ribbon, and extra-absorbent versions with an adhesive backing. A major advantage of these products is that they can be removed without causing pain to the client.

Alginate dressings vary in both their chemical and physical properties. Therefore, it is essential that prior to the selection of a product, a wound assessment be undertaken. It is important that this assessment takes into consideration both the size and condition of the wound, along with the individual needs of the client. For example, if the client's environmental and social situation allows bathing, *Kaltoclude*® and *Sorbsan SA*® are water-proof and can be worn whilst in the bath.

Certain alginates will cause maceration and excoriation of surrounding skin. Therefore, particular attention must be paid when applying these products. If using *Kaltostat*®, the dressing should be cut or folded to fit flat wounds correctly. An important point to remember when applying algi-nate dressings, is that they must be covered with a secondary dressing to conserve moisture. Failure to do so will result in the alginate drying out. The selection of the secondary dressing will depend on the quantity of exudate. In situations where exudate is copious, absorbent pads are effec-tive. However, if exudate is minimal, a vapour-permeable film dressing can be used.

Alginates are biodegradable. However, it is important when removing the dressing, that any remaining traces are removed from the wound. Irrigation with 0.9% sodium chloride solution will dissolve *Sorbsan*® and *Kaltogel*®. However, *Tegagen*® and *Kaltostat*® are less soluble. Therefore, these dress-ings need to be soaked in 0.9% sodium chloride prior to removal. They can then be removed intact from the wound.

It is possible to leave alginate dressing products in place for 7 days although, ideally, they should be removed after they have been *in situ* for 3-5 days. In circumstances where wounds have large amounts of exudate, manufacturers recommend that dressings be changed daily. However, if appropriate secondary dressings are selected, they will absorb the exudate, which will prevent interrupting the moist wound environment. *Kaltostat Fortex®* sheets are also very effective in heavily exuding wounds. This product has increased absorbent capacity, which will allow fewer dressing changes. In situations where wounds are infected, daily dressing changes should be considered.

**Table 7.2** summarises the different types of wounds and describes the appropriate dressing types.

## Desloughing agents

Streptokinase and Streptodornase Topical Powder is a desloughing agent available in the NPF.

## Mode of action

This preparation activates a fibrinolytic enzyme in human serum. The activation of this system causes rapid dissolution of blood clots and the fibrinous portion of exudates. Dead cells or puss are liquefied. These actions facilitate the cleansing and desloughing of wounds.

## Indications for use

Streptokinase and Streptodornase Topical Powder is indicated in the treatment of suppurative surface lesions such as ulcers, pressure sores, amputa-

**Table 7.2** - *Wound type and appropriate dressing*

| Wound Type | Type of Dressing |
|---|---|
| Dry, necrotic wounds | Hydrocolloids and Hydrogels |
| Slough-covered wounds | Hydrocolloids and Hydrogels |
| Clean, exuding wounds (granulating) | Hydrocolloids, Foams, Alginates |
| Clean, dry, low exudate wounds (epithelialising) | Absorbent Perforated Plastic Film-Faced Dressing |
| | Vapour-permeable Adhesive film dressings |
| Clean, medium-to-high exudate wounds (epithelialising) | Knitted Varicose Primary Dressing Paraffin gauze |

tion sites, diabetic gangrene, radiation necrosis, infected wounds and surgical incisions.

## Administration

Reconstitute with 20 ml sterile physiological saline or water for injection and apply as a wet dressing 1–2 times daily. A semi-occlusive dressing should be used to cover the lesion. Between applications the lesion should be irrigated thoroughly with physiological saline and any loosened material removed.

---

**CONTRA-INDICATIONS**

Active haemorrhage

**SIDE-EFFECTS**

Allergic reactions are infrequent and can be minimised by the careful and frequent removal of exudate, followed by thorough irrigation with physiological saline. Transient slight burning pain has been reported.

---

## Bandages

Products in the NPF range from Cotton Conforming Bandages used in the retention of dressings, to compression bandages applied to chronic leg ulcers. It is important to appreciate that the outer layers of a dressing are important for a number of reasons including:

- The provision of support for the wound and surrounding tissue.
- The maintenance of the position of the dressing.
- The absorption of moisture.
- The control of oedema.
- To act as a splint.

Whichever dressing is selected, it is important to appreciate that the elastic properties of a bandage determine its ability to support or compress the wound and retain a dressing. The tension of the application of the bandage, the bandage width, and the radius of the limb, will determine the pressure beneath the bandage. When selecting an appropriate outer layer or bandage the hazards of inappropriate or excessive pressure must be realised. In situations where perfusion pressures are low (i.e. arterial ulcers), compression should not be applied, as the capillary bed may collapse resulting in further tissue damage. By contrast, in venous ulceration, external pressure applied from ankle to knee is advocated, in order to reduce venous pooling.

## References

Bux, M. (1996). Selection and use of wound dressings. *Wound Care for Pharmacists* Summer issue: 11–16.

Dealey, C. (1994). *The Care of Wounds*. Oxford: Blackwell Scientific Publications.

Dunford, C. (1997). Management of recurrent pilonidal sinus. *Nursing Times* 93(32): 64.

Thomas, S. (1990). *Wound Management and Dressings*. London: The Pharmaceutical Press.

Winter, G.D. (1962). Formation of the scab and the rate of epithelialisation of superficial wounds in the skin of the young domestic pig. *Nature* 193: 293–294.

# 8

# CATHETER MANAGEMENT PREPARATIONS

The NPF (see **Appendix 2**) lists several preparations required for urinary catheter management. These include local anaesthetic agents, necessary for insertion of urinary catheters, and catheter patency solutions. These products will be considered, together with their mode of action and relevant nursing points.

## LOCAL ANAESTHESIA

### Applied anatomy and physiology

In order to sense pain or discomfort, receptors must be stimulated and nerve impulses must be sent to the central nervous system (see **Chapter 5**). Conduction of a nerve impulse involves a rapid series of events occuring both inside and outside the nerve cell membrane.

A neurone that is not conducting a nerve impulse is said to be "resting". The cell membrane of the "resting" neurone is said to be polarised. This means that the intracellular fluid on the inside of the membrane is electrically charged in relation to the charged extracellular fluid outside the membrane. The difference in the charge between the inside and the outside of the cell membrane is called the potential difference. The potential difference across the membrane of a resting neurone is called the resting membrane potential. It is due to the unequal distribution of ions and the permeability of the ion channels located in the cell membrane. Sodium ions are in a higher concentration in the extracellular fluid, whilst potassium ions are in a higher concentration inside the cell. There are channels for both of these ions, present in the cell membrane.

It is the change in the potential difference across the membrane that is the key factor in the initiation and conduction of a nerve impulse. A stimulus strong enough to initiate a nerve impulse is called a threshold stimulus. When the threshold stimulus is applied to the resting neuronal membrane, sodium channels open and sodium rushes into the cell. This reverses the electrical charge, with the inside of the membrane having a positive charge relative to the outside of the membrane, at the point of stimulus. This process is referred to as depolarisation. Once a small area on the nerve axon is depolarised, it then stimulates an adjacent area which also contains ion channels. Thus a nerve impulse or, more specifically, an action potential, is initiated, which passes along the neuronal cell membrane. After depolarisation has occured, the original balance of sodium and potassium ions has to be restored, as sodium has entered the cell and some potassium has left the cell via open potassium channels. This is carried out by the sodium-potassium pump found within the cell membrane, which transports two potassium ions back into the nerve cell for every three sodium ions that it transfers out. This ensures the relative negative charge inside the resting cell, and the relative positive charge outside the cell. The cell membrane is now said to be repolarised.

## Mode of action of local anaesthetics

Local anaesthetics such as lignocaine are used to prevent pain and discomfort. They cause a reversible block of conduction along nerve fibres to produce both a loss of sensation and a loss of muscle activity. Small, non-myelinated pain fibres are most sensitive to these drugs, and are the first to be depressed. Subsequent loss of function of other types of nerves occurs, in the following order: temperature, touch, proprioception, and skeletal muscle tone (Pinnell, 1996).

The drug is administered at the desired site of action. It will penetrate the nerve axon and bind to receptors in the sodium channels (**Figure 8.1**). This results in blocking of the sodium channels. Ultimately, many channels become blocked and depolarisation of the cell membrane is not possible. Action potentials cannot be generated and the nerve becomes 'blocked'. The inhibition of nerve conduction will persist until the drug diffuses, and enters the circulation for subsequent metabolism and excretion.

The duration of the block is increased if adrenaline (epinephrine) is incorporated into the preparation. Adrenaline will cause vasoconstriction and therefore reduce systemic absorption of the local anaesthetic. Adrenaline is, however, contraindicated for infiltration of areas with end arteries (fingers, toes, ears, nose, penis). Ischaemia may occur, resulting in death of the tissue concerned (Clark *et al*, 1997). None of the NPF preparations contain adrenaline.

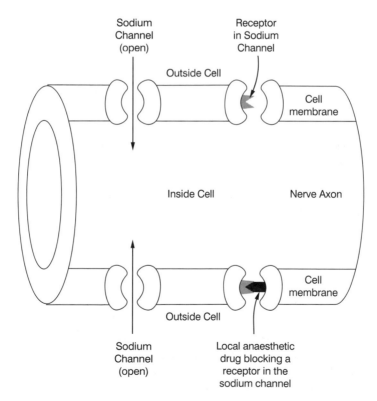

*Figure 8.1* – Local anaesthetic drug blocking a sodium channel.

## Preparations in the NPF

- **Lignocaine gel** (*Xylocaine*® gel)

- **Lignocaine ointment** (*Xylocaine*® ointment)

- **Lignocaine and chlorhexidine gel** (*Xylocaine*® antiseptic gel)

The NPF preparations are all topical or surface anaesthetics. These are used for anaesthetising the skin and mucous membranes. They may be required during clinical examination, catheterisation, for minor burns or abrasions, and local symptomatic relief of pain. Intact skin is penetrated poorly, whilst broken skin and mucous membranes allow more rapid absorption of the drug. Lignocaine is the most widely used of all local anaesthetics. It acts rapidly and is more stable than most of the other available drugs. Onset of action occurs within 3-5 minutes with the duration of action being approximately 1.0-1.5 hours.

---

### CONTRAINDICATIONS

Caution should be taken if the client has a history of epilepsy, hepatic impairment or cardiac disease. Care should be taken in infants and young children and there is risk of choking if used in the mouth.

### SIDE-EFFECTS

Skin rash, due to local allergy, may occur with chronic use. Excessive application may result in increased absorption and systemic side-effects. These may include convulsions, paraesthesia, nervousness, tremors, hypotension and bradycardia.

---

## Nursing points

*Use of an anaesthetic gel for urinary catheterisation is common practice, and will reduce both pain and trauma on insertion of the catheter. In practice, it is often only men who require a lubricating, anaesthetic gel inserted prior to catheterisation (Mackenzie & Webb, 1995). The use of a gel is, however, advocated for women as well as men (Mackenzie & Webb, 1995; de Courcy-Ireland, 1993).*

*Usually, 10 ml is inserted into the male urethra and this may be followed by a further 5 ml. Women may require 5-10 ml prior to catheterisation.*

*Clients requiring a local anaesthetic to be applied to the skin should be educated about not exceeding the recommended dose and should also be made familiar with potential side-effects of excessive absorption.*

# CATHETER PATENCY SOLUTIONS

Many nurse prescribers will be involved in the care of clients with long term, indwelling, urinary catheters. Several complications are associated with the use of catheters, including catheter blockage, catheter encrustation, inflammatory reactions, trauma, urine infection, pain and discomfort. Winn, (1998) and Kunin *et al* (1987) report that approximately 50 per cent of all patients with an indwelling catheter are prone to catheter blockage, which occurs secondary to encrustation. In addition, blocked catheters may cause bypassing or retention of urine.

## Encrustation

In alkaline conditions, ammonium phosphate, calcium phosphate or magnesium phosphate may precipitate from the urine and collect on the tip or around the eyes or the balloon of the catheter. In addition, infected urine is also more likely to lead to encrustation. The presence of bacteria such as *Proteus, Klebsiella* and *Pseudomonas* specifically encourages the process of encrustation (Getliffe, 1997). It is the release of urease enzyme from these micro-organisms which breaks down urea to release ammonia and hydrogen ions, hence causing an increase in urine alkalinity.

The presence of a biofilm on the surface of the catheter also increases the risk of infection, encrustation and associated problems (Ramsey, 1989). A biofilm is a collection of micro-organisms and their products on a solid surface (Wilson, 1998). Bacteria within the biofilm produce a glycocalyx or thick coat of polysaccharides. This coat protects the micro-organism from the body's natural defence mechanisms and antimicrobial drugs.

## Catheter material

The type of catheter material may have some effect on the development of encrustation and development of a biofilm. Winn (1998) reports the results of several studies that indicate that all-silicone catheters are less likely to become encrusted than silicone-coated, Teflon-coated and latex catheters over 14 days. Hydrogel-coated catheters appear to be as resistant to encrustation as all-silicone catheters over a period up to 18 weeks. In addition, hydrogel-coated catheters are less prone to bacterial adherence than silicone catheters. However, the ideal catheter, resisting encrustation and biofilm development, is not yet available, and nurses need to be aware of the specific characteristics of products in order to make an informed choice about which appliance to choose for their client.

## Catheter life

Getliffe (1996) suggests that observing and recording the length of time that a client's catheter continues to function before becoming blocked, will reveal a pattern of 'catheter life'. It should then be possible to plan future recatheterisations before blockage has a chance to recur.

In addition, the reduction of urine alkalinity by consumption of cranberry juice may assist in prolonging catheter life. The resulting acidification of urine may prevent infection and encrustation. Busuttil Leaver (1996) identifies some of the potential effects of cranberry juice but more research is required.

If a client experiences no problems with blockage, the catheter needs to be changed approximately 3 monthly if all-silicone, silicone-coated or hydrogel-coated. Latex catheters require changing every 6 weeks in most instances. Frequent blocking, however, requires either recatheterisation, which can be painful if it is being done often, or the use of an appropriate bladder washout solution to attempt to relieve the obstruction.

Catheter maintenance solutions in the NPF include:

- **Chlorhexidene 0.02%** (*Uro-Tainer Chlorhexidene®*, *Uriflex C®*)

- **Mandelic Acid 1%** (*Uro-Tainer Mandelic Acid®*)

- **Sodium Chloride 0.9%** (*Uro-Tainer Sodium Chloride®*, *Uriflex S®*)

- **'Solution G'** (*Uro-Tainer Suby G®*, *Uriflex G®*)

- **'Solution R'** (*Uro-Tainer Solution R®*, *Uriflex R®*)

Chlorhexidene 0.02% solution is available for mechanical cleansing and prevention of contamination by bacteria, specifically *Escherichia coli* and *Klebsiella*. It is usually ineffective against most species of *Pseudomonas*. Mandelic acid 1% aids acidification in order to prevent growth of urease-producing bacteria, as well as mechanically cleansing the catheter and bladder. Sodium chloride 0.9% will aid small blood clot removal and tissue debris that may be present. 'Solution G' specifically prevents encrustation and crystallisation. 'Solution R' is recommended for prevention of encrustation and crystallisation when 'Solution G' has been unsuccessful.

---

### SIDE-EFFECTS

Chlorhexidene 0.02% may irritate the bladder causing burning and haematuria. Its should be discontinued in these circumstances.

---

## Nursing points

*The use of a catheter maintenance solution requires the breaking of a closed drainage system. Aseptic technique must, therefore, be performed when administering a solution. A new drainage bag should be connected following the procedure. Hands should be washed thoroughly before and after the procedure.*

*The solution should be warmed to body temperature before instillation. Gravity is used to instill the solution and not active flushing.*

*Ideally, bladder washouts should only be used when absolutely necessary. However, prophylactic washouts in clients with frequently blocked catheters may extend the catheter life.*

*Clients and/or their carers can be taught to administer a catheter patency solution. Client or carer assessment is essential in order to establish that they have the manual dexterity and ability to undertake their own catheter management. A planned teaching programme will be necessary to help them develop confidence and competence in catheter care (Getliffe, 1996).*

*Clients should be encouraged to maintain an adequate fluid intake to reduce the irritant effects of concentrated urine and maintain urine flow. An intake of 1.5-2.0 litres per day is recommended. A high fluid intake cannot prevent or reduce infection, but diuresis may assist in voiding micro-organisms from the bladder.*

*If clients wish to consume cranberry juice, then the nurse should attempt to monitor its effects on the client. No more than one litre per day should be consumed, as an excessive intake may lead to uric acid stone formation. Clients with irritable bowel syndrome may develop diarrhoea. In addition, cranberry juice is rather expensive and some individuals will dislike its taste.*

# References

Busuttil Leaver R. (1996). Cranberry juice. *Professional Nurse* May; 11(8): 525–526.

Clarke J.B., Queener S.F. and Karb V.(1997). *Pharmacologic Basis of Nursing Practice* (5ᵗʰ edition). St Louis: Mosby.

de Courcy-Ireland K. (1993). An issue of sensitivity: use of analgesic gel in catheterising women. *Professional Nurse* 8(11): 738–742.

Getliffe K. (1996). Care of urinary catheters. *Nursing Standard* 11(11): 47–50.

Getliffe K. (1997). Catheters and catheterisation. In: Getliffe K., Dolman M. (eds). *Promoting Continence: A Clinical and Research Resource*. London: Balliere Tindall.

Kunin C.M., Chin Q.F. and Chambers S. (1987). Formation of encrustations on indwelling urinary catheters in the elderly: a comparison of different types of catheter materials in 'blockers' and 'non-blockers'. *Journal of Urology* 138(4): 899–902.

Mackenzie J. and Webb C. (1995). Gynopia in nursing practice: the case of urethral catheterisation. *Journal of Clinical Nursing* 4: 221–226.

Ramsey J. (1989). Biofilms, bacteria and bladder catheters – a clinical study. *British Journal of Urology* 64: 395–398.

Wilson M. (1998). Infection control. *Professional Nurse Study Supplement* February, 13 (5), S10-S13.

Winn C. (1998). Complications with urinary catheters. *Professional Nurse Study Supplement* February, 13(5): S7–10.

# 9

# ORAL AND EAR PREPARATIONS

Preparations to treat fungal infection of the mouth may now be prescribed by the nurse practitioner. In addition, two products used for the softening of ear wax are also listed in the NPF (**Appendix 2**). All of these preparations will be considered in this chapter, together with the relevant information from the biological sciences to support and inform practice.

## ORAL PREPARATIONS

These products include antifungal medications to treat oral candidiasis and a simple mouthwash solution for general cleansing or the management of traumatic ulceration.

### Fungal infection of the mouth

Fungi that do not usually cause disease may do so in individuals who have altered body defence mechanisms. These fungi are referred to as 'opportunists'. *Candida albicans* is a yeast-like, opportunistic fungus (**Figure 9.1**)

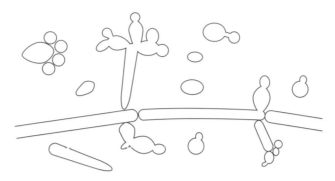

**Figure 9.1** – *Candida albicans*. Hyphae giving rise to budding yeast-like cells.

that is responsible for approximately 90% of all *Candida* infections, and causes the most common of all oral fungal infections.

*C. albicans* is part of the normal flora of the mouth, intestine and vagina of humans. However, it is responsible for infection in these sites when local conditions are disrupted or defence mechanisms become impaired. Areas affected are mainly the mucosae where *C. albicans* is normally present in health, and on regions of moist skin. The infection is more commonly referred to as 'thrush'.

Clients most susceptible to opportunistic *C. albicans* include:

- pregnant women
- debilitated infants
- elderly people
- those with immunodeficiency (eg. clients with AIDS, clients receiving cancer chemotherapy)
- those having received antibiotic or corticosteroid therapy
- those with indwelling urinary or intravenous catheters
- those with diabetes mellitus                         (Brooks *et al*, 1991)

The most common sites for *C. albicans* infection are the vagina and mouth. Preparations listed in the NPF allow the nurse prescriber to treat oral *Candida* and *Candida* infection of the skin and genital region (see **Chapter 4**). The oral condition is usually diagnosed following the observation of creamy white patches covering raw areas of mucous membrane and tongue within the buccal cavity. An oral swab, taken for culture and sensitivity, will provide laboratory confirmation of the infection. Diagnosis is easily made on detection of large, Gram-positive, budding yeasts (Mims *et al*, 1993).

*C. albicans* occurs particularly in adults with inflammation of the corners of the mouth (angular cheilitis), ill-fitting dentures, those adults that have had prolonged antibiotic therapy and those who are immunocompromised.

In infants, the infection may be difficult to distinguish from coagulated milk lining the buccal cavity. Diagnosis, however, is usually apparent when attempts to remove white patches with a spatula are unsuccessful. The source of the infection in the newborn is usually from maternal vaginal infection. The infant or child may also acquire the infection from contaminated hands, bottles, teats, nipples or other articles (Wong, 1997). The infection may cause refusal to feed and may also be accompanied by fever and gastrointestinal irritation. It commonly spreads to the groin and buttocks (McCance & Huether, 1994) and these lesions should be treated with a local antifungal drug (see **Chapter 4**).

### Treatment

It is important before treating the infection, to try and identify the circumstances that may have lead to the infection. If the underlying problem can be corrected, for example by improving oral hygiene or controlling blood glucose in diabetes mellitus, then the body may well be able to deal with the infection. However, treatment will shorten this process.

The three preparations to treat oral *C. albicans* are:

- **Miconazole oral gel** (*Daktarin*® oral gel)
- **Nystatin pastilles** (*Nystan*® pastilles)
- **Nystatin oral suspension** (*Nystan*® oral suspension)

Miconazole belongs to the imidazole group of anti-fungal agents. It is a broad spectrum drug which acts by inhibiting ergosterol synthesis in the fungal cell membrane. Ergosterol is a major constituent of the fungal cell membrane, and thus fungal growth is prevented by miconazole. Nystatin however, binds to ergosterol molecules in the fungal cell membrane which alters membrane permeability and hence allows leakage of intracellular contents.

There is minimal absorption of nystatin after oral administration, with most of the drug being eliminated in faeces.

## CONTRAINDICATIONS

The contraindications for miconazole are hepatic impairment and previous hypersensitivity to the drug. It should be used with caution in pregnancy. It increases the activity of some other drugs when taken at the same time. These include anticoagulants (warfarin), antidiabetics (sulphonylureas) and antiepileptics (phenytoin). It antagonises the effects of the antifungal drug, amphotericin.

The only contraindication for the use of nystatin is a previous history of allergic reaction on exposure to the drug.

## SIDE-EFFECTS

Nystatin is usually well tolerated by individuals of all age groups. Some individuals may get some oral irritation. Large doses may cause nausea, diarrhoea and vomiting.

Oral miconazole may produce mild gastrointestinal upset. Nausea, vomiting and diarrhoea may occur if used for long periods. Allergy only occurs rarely.

## Nursing points

*In adults, miconazole gel 5-10 ml should be applied 6 hourly for 10 days, or for up to 2 days after the symptoms have cleared. Children over 6 years of age require 5 ml, 4 times daily whilst children under 2 years are prescribed 2.5 ml twice daily. The gel is applied after food and should be retained in the mouth for as long as possible. Clients require information about hand hygiene. Hands should be washed before and after application. Contact with the eyes and nose should be avoided when applying miconazole.*

*The dose of nystatin for both adults and children is the same. The dose of the oral suspension is 100,000U (1 ml) 4 times daily after food, or one pastille 4 times daily after food. Clients with immunosuppression may need higher doses up to 500,000U 4 times daily. Those taking the oral suspension should be instructed to place 0.5 ml inside each cheek, and then keep in the mouth for as long as possible before swallowing. Nystatin should be continued for 2 days after the infection has resolved. As for miconazole, good hand hygiene is important.*

*Clients with dental prostheses, that have oral C. albicans infection, should soak them in chlorhexidene for ten minutes in order to reduce the risk of reinfecting the mouth with contaminated dentures (Mallet and Bailey, 1996).*

*Measures to control C. albicans in infants and children include: rinsing the infant's mouth with plain water after each feed and before applying medication; sterilisation of feeding bottles, teats and pacifiers. Infants with candidal nappy dermatitis can introduce yeast into the mouth from contaminated hands. The placing of clothing over the nappy can prevent the cycle of re-infection (Wong, 1997).*

*Clients should be encouraged to take the preparation for the prescribed period.*

### Thymol glycerin

The nurse may prescribe this product for clients that require a general mouthwash to freshen the mouth, or to assist in the relief of pain from traumatic ulceration. The mouth wash is diluted with warm water and used as required for general oral hygiene. It may be used at frequent intervals until the discomfort and inflammation of ulceration subsides.

## EAR PREPARATIONS

### Applied anatomy and physiology of the ear

The ear is divided into three main parts; the external ear, middle ear and inner ear (**Figure 9.2**). The external ear consists of the pinna, external auditory meatus (ear canal) and tympanic membrane (eardrum).

The pinna is the large, skin-covered flap of cartilage which collects sound waves and channels them into and down the external auditory meatus. It also protects the opening of the external auditory meatus. In the adult, the external auditory meatus is approximately 2.5 cm long and its entrance is guarded by fine hairs.

The skin lining this canal contains wax-secreting ceruminous glands, which are modified sebaceous glands. The earwax or cerumen, consists of the secretion of the ceruminous glands, together with desquamated epithelial cells shed from the skin lining the canal, and variable amounts of hair. It functions to trap foreign objects and insects, and to slow the growth of

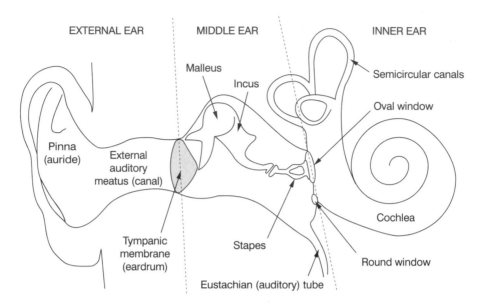

***Figure 9.2*** – Anatomy of the ear.

microorganisms in the ear canal. The presence of immunoglobulins and lysosymes, together with the skin of the ear being approximately pH 6.0, is thought to assist in defence against invading micro-organisms (Li Wan Po, 1990). Cerumen also prevents the skin of the external ear from drying out. Both the hairs and earwax will reduce the chance of airborne particles from reaching the inner part of the ear canal where they may accumulate and interfere with hearing.

The ear canal ends at the tympanic membrane which stretches across the entrance to the middle ear.

This thin, semi-transparent membrane vibrates when struck by sound waves that have been directed along the ear canal. The air-filled middle ear then transfers the vibratory movements of the tympanic membrane to the fluid of the inner ear. Three small bones (the malleus, incus and stapes), also called the auditory ossicles, facilitate the transfer of vibrations through the middle ear. The stapes is attached to the oval window which bows in and out as the stapes moves back and forth. Movement of the oval window causes waves to occur in the fluid of the cochlea. A further series of events in the inner ear ultimately leads to the interpretation of sound by the central nervous system. For a fuller discussion of this process the reader should refer to Martini (1998).

## Conductive hearing loss

There are several reasons why sound waves may not be transmitted to the inner ear. These include blockage of the external auditory meatus, infection of the middle ear, perforation of the tympanic membrane and immobilisation of one or more of the auditory ossicles. These conditions in the external and middle ear prevent the normal transfer of vibrations from the tympanic membrane to the oval window. This results in difficulties with hearing, referred to as conductive hearing loss (conductive deafness).

The most common cause of partial, conductive hearing loss is the accumulation of earwax in the external auditory meatus. Normally, wax migrates naturally to the outside of the external meatus but this process may be hindered. If ear hairs are tough (as in elderly males), or if the client attempts to clean the ears by poking a cotton wool bud down the canal, the wax may simply be pushed in the wrong direction. Not infrequently, the wax may become impacted in the canal, where, over time, it becomes hard (Serra *et al*, 1986). As earwax is a normal body secretion with protective functions, it should only be removed if it is causing hearing problems or interfering with a view of the eardrum on examination. Excessive wax or blockage by wax may be treated by instilling ear drops to soften the wax, or by ear syringing with warm water.

NPF preparations available as ear drops are:

- **Almond oil ear drops**
- **Olive oil ear drops**

These preparations may be referred to as ceruminolytics as they soften and loosen excessive or impacted wax (cerumen).

---

### CONTRAINDICATIONS

The nurse prescriber should avoid prescribing ear drops to: clients with a history of ear disease, to all cases of earache, and clients complaining of dizziness or an ear discharge. It is advisable to refer the client to their General Practitioner for further assessment.

### SIDE-EFFECTS

These are not common. Minor skin irritation may occur.

---

## Nursing points

*Ear drops should be warmed prior to instillation. This is best achieved by holding the bottle of oil in the hand for 5-10 minutes, allowing the temperature of the preparation to rise to body temperature. The client should lie with the affected ear uppermost. A reasonable amount of oil is introduced into the ear and the client should remain in the same position for 5-10 minutes to enable softening of the wax. The client or carer will need to be instructed about administration of the ear drops. If ear syringing is required, following wax softening using ear drops, it should only be undertaken by a proficient practitioner, trained in the procedure.*

*Mechanical probing of the ears with implements such as cotton buds, hair pins and matchsticks should be discouraged. This only serves to enhance blockage by wax and could possibly perforate the eardrum. Baxter (1983) recommends that cerumi-nolytics are safer than cotton buds.*

# References

Baxter P. (1983). Association between the use of cotton tipped swabs and cerumen plugs. *British Medical Journal* 287: 1260.

Brooks G.F., Butel J.S., Ornston L.N., Jawetz E., Melnick J.L. and Adelberg E.A. (1991). *Medical Microbiology* (19th edition). Norwalk: Appleton and Lange.

Li Wan Po A. (1990). *Non-Prescription Drugs* (2nd edition). Oxford: Blackwell Scientific Publications.

McCance K.L. and Huether S.E. (1994). *Pathophysiology: The Biologic Basis of Disease in Adults and Children* (2nd edition). St. Louis: Mosby.

Mallet J. and Bailey C. (1996). *The Royal Marsden NHS Trust Manual of Clinical Nursing Procedures* (4th ed.). Oxford: Blackwell Science.

Martini F.H. (1998). *Fundamentals of Anatomy and Physiology* (4th edition). New Jersey: Prentice Hall.

Mims C.A., Playfair J.H.L., Roitt I.M., Wakelin D., Williams R. and Anderson R.M. (1993). *Medical Microbiology* St Louis: Mosby.

Serra A.M., Bailey C.M. and Jackson P. (1986). *Ear, Nose and Throat Nursing.* Oxford: Blackwell Scientific Publications.

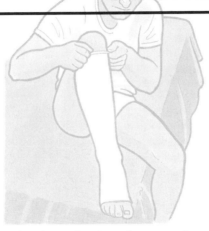

# 10

# ELASTIC HOSIERY

The nurse will prescribe elastic hosiery for a number of conditions including, the prevention and treatment of varicose veins and leg ulcers, the control of oedema, and the prevention of deep vein thrombosis (DVT). This chapter commences with an overview of the circulatory system including the respiratory and venous pump systems. The role of graduated compression and elastic hosiery on blood flow, venous pressure and oedema is then examined. A description of the different classes, styles, and types of elastic hosiery follow this. Measuring and fitting elastic hosiery and the care of these garments is then discussed.

## THE CIRCULATORY SYSTEM

Blood flows through the body in a closed network called the circulatory system. From the left ventricle, blood passes into the aorta and then into other arteries. Arteries carry the blood away from the heart. Each artery branches approximately fifteen to twenty times, becoming smaller and smaller. These small arteries are called arterioles, which lead into a network of minute capillaries. Oxygen and nutrients diffuse through the thin walls of these vessels into the tissues of the body. The capillaries eventually form venules, which lead onto veins. Veins take the blood back to the right atrium. The right ventricle then pumps this blood to the lungs where it becomes oxygenated, and then it returns to the left side of the heart. The blood therefore has two journeys: around the body in the systemic circulation, and to the lungs and back in the pulmonary circulation. At any one time, three quarters of the blood is in veins, one fifth in arteries, and one-twentieth in capillaries.

## The structure of blood vessels

Arteries and veins are composed of three layers:

- *Tunica adventia*: This layer is the outermost layer of the vessel and forms a connective tissue sheath. This sheath helps to stabilise and anchor the vessel by the blending of connective tissue fibres into adjacent tissue. In veins, the tunica adventia is generally thicker than the tunica media.

- *Tunica media*: This layer consists of involuntary muscle, which is stimulated by sympathetic nerve fibres, and elastic fibres. It is responsible for the change in lumen size of the vessel, and is very thick in arteries. In vasodilation, the muscle is relaxed and the vessel open. In vasoconstriction, the muscle contracts, and the vessel narrows. Collagen fibres within the tunica media bind it to the tunica adventia and tunica intima.

- *Tunica intima*: This layer is comprised of a smooth lining of endothelial cells, which also forms the valves, and a basement membrane.

Blood vessels are designed in such a way as to function effectively in their specific roles (**Figure 10.1**). Capillaries are comprised of a single layer of cells, and so allow the easy passage of oxygen and nutrients into the surrounding tissue. Arteries have very thick muscular walls, enabling them to cope with the high-pressure surges of blood from the heart. Veins have loose, slack walls as the blood in them is under very little pressure.

## Venous return

The pressure in the venous system determines the volume of blood returned to the heart. This is directly related to cardiac output and periph-

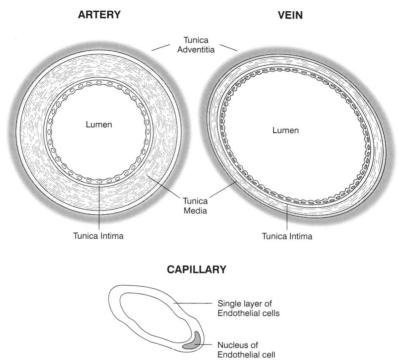

**ARTERY**

**VEIN**

Tunica
Adventitia

Lumen

Lumen

Tunica
Media

Tunica Intima

Tunica Intima

**CAPILLARY**

Single layer of
Endothelial cells

Nucleus of
Endothelial cell

*Figure 10.1* – The structure of blood vessels.

eral blood flow. To maintain cardiac output, the venous blood has to travel through a complex vascular network. However, the blood pressure at the beginning of the venous system is approximately ten times less than at the start of the arterial system.

Three input mechanisms are involved in the return of the venous blood to the heart:

- The respiratory pump.
- The venous pump.
- Venous valves.

### The respiratory pump

The thoracic cavity expands as a person inhales and the pressure within the pleural cavities are reduced. This drop in pressure causes air to be pulled into the lungs. At the same time, blood is also pulled from the smaller veins of the abdominal cavity and lower body into the inferior vena cava and right atrium. During exhalation, the thoracic cavity is decreased in size. Thus the internal pressure is caused to rise. Air is forced out of the lungs, and venous blood pushed into the right atrium.

## The venous pump

The venous system of the leg (**Figure 10.2**), comprises:

- The femoral, popliteal, and tibial deep veins encased and supported by the tough, deep fascia muscle sheath.

- The long and short saphenous superficia veins lying outside the fascia.

- The short perforator connecting veins perforate the fascia.

The pressure of the blood in the leg veins results from the weight of the blood itself and is highest at the lowest point. When an individual is standing still, the pressure of the blood in the deep veins of the foot is approximately 90 mmHg. This pressure is much lower in the superficial veins and capillaries.

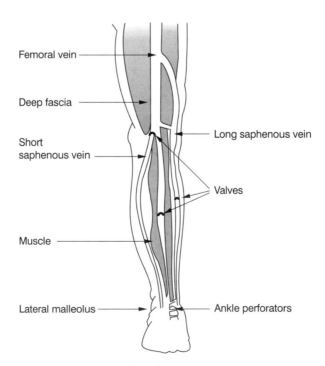

*Figure 10.2* – The venous system of the leg.

During normal standing and walking, the venous pump assists venous return. As the calf muscles contract, they become shorter and thicker and compress nearby blood vessels propelling blood towards the heart. During muscle relaxation, the vessel once again fills with blood and the cycle is repeated during the next contraction. When a person is standing still for a long period of time, the venous pump does not operate and blood pools in the legs.

### Venous valves

The valves, present in leg veins, play a crucial role in the efficiency of the venous pump. Valves are formed from the endothelial lining of the tunica intima and are semi-lunar folds that point in the direction of blood flow. The valves in the leg veins have a similar action to the valves in the heart. They allow blood to flow in one direction only, and prevent it from flowing back towards the capillaries. Therefore, any movement that distorts or compresses a vein will push blood towards the heart. Without valves, the effects of gravity when standing upright would cause pooling of blood in the leg veins and fail to overcome the pull of gravity to ascend to the heart.

The blood is compartmentalised by valves. Therefore, the weight of the blood is divided between each of the compartments in the vein. Movement in the surrounding skeletal muscle squeezes the blood towards the heart. When standing, very fast cycles of contraction and relaxation occur within the leg muscles, the contractions pushing the blood towards the heart. When lying down, the heart and major vessels are at the same level. Therefore, venous valves have much less impact on venous return.

The valves in the perforator connecting veins have the most important role. If these valves fail to work effectively, the high pressure in the deep veins, is transmitted to the much weaker, unsupported superficial veins. These veins become distended and tortuous (varicose veins). Capillary pressure becomes increased, and fluid is forced out into the extravascular space. This can then progress onto chronic venous insufficiency characterised by oedema, pigmentation, eczema, and ulceration of the leg.

## GRADUATED COMPRESSION THERAPY

Graduated compression therapy plays a major role in the treatment and prevention of varicose veins and leg ulcers, the control of oedema, and the prevention of deep vein thrombosis (DVT). This therapy works by providing pressure and support for the superficial vessels. This counteracts the raised capillary pressure and prevents oedema.

Graded compression stockings exert a greater pressure at the toe than at the thigh. This therefore, provides a constant graded pressure and encourages the complete emptying of veins, decreasing venous pooling and venous stasis.

The amount of pressure required will depend on the size of the patient's leg and the severity of the disease. However, ideally, the pressure should be no greater than that required to prevent capillary leakage.

## Categories of compression hosiery

A range of elastic hosiery is specified by the British Standards Institution (BSI). Stockings are classified according to the maximum pressure at the ankle and the pressure gradients at calf and thigh (**Figure 10.3**). Standard methods are in place for batch testing of these garments, and an important attribute is durability. Stockings have to maintain 85% of their original pressure after 30 washes in accordance with the manufacturer's instructions.

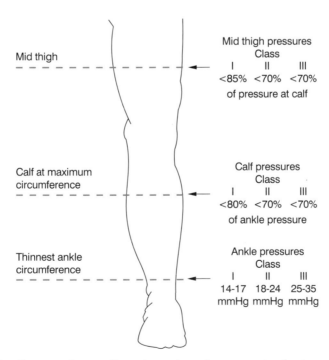

*Figure 10.3* – Compression gradients in graduated compression hosiery.

## Classes

There are three different classes of compression hosiery. Each class differs with regard to the level of pressure exerted. The classes, as described by the Drug Tariff (1998), are as follows:

**Class I:** This class provides light (mild) support and produces compression of 14 mmHg – 17 mmHg at the ankle.

*Indications:* These stockings are for superficial or early varices and those occurring during pregnancy.

**Class II:** These stockings provide medium (moderate) support. Compression at the ankle is 18 mmHg – 24 mmHg.

*Indications:* They are generally used for: varices of medium severity, ulcer treatment and prevention of recurrence, mild oedema, varicosis during pregnancy, and for soft tissue support.

**Class III:** These stockings provide strong support. Compression at the ankle is 25 mmHg – 35 mmHg.

*Indications:* This class is used for: gross varices, post thrombotic venous insufficiency, gross oedema, ulcer treatment and prevention of recurrence, and soft tissue support.

## Types

There are several types of compression stocking. These include:

### Circular knit stockings

These stockings are available in cotton and nylon yarn. The modern stockings use elastane as opposed to rubber and are cosmetically more acceptable. A disadvantage with these stockings is a lack of stretch. This makes them very difficult to put on particularly for the elderly client.

### Flat bed knit stockings

These can be obtained in cotton, nylon, and nylon-plated varieties. The nylon-plated variety are the most durable, whilst the nylon has the least ankle pressure, and the cotton can be the most comfortable. These stockings are made from welt to toe and have a fashioning line down the back. They tend to be more flexible than circular knit stockings and are easier to put on and take off. Therefore, they may be more preferable for people with swollen legs, those with arthritis, and the elderly. Flat bed knit stockings are only available as a made-to-measure item on prescription only.

### Net stockings

These types of stockings are often the least cosmetically acceptable. They are made out of a net fabric and seamed. Net stockings are also only available as a made-to-measure item.

### One – way stretch stockings (Class III only)

These stockings are made to measure in a very heavy circular machine knit. They are seamless apart from the finishing at the toe and the heel.

## Style

Thigh length, below knee stockings, socks and tights are all styles of compression hosiery available. Each item conforms to the British Standard Compression requirement and come in made to measure and standard sizes. Manufacturers also offer different combinations of colour and open or closed heels or toes.

## THE SELECTION OF COMPRESSION HOSIERY

The style of stocking should be determined in the initial assessment. A number of factors influence the type and style of stocking selected. These include:

- The client's age.
- The dexterity of the client.
- Whether or not the client is disabled.
- The condition of the client's skin.
- The appearance of the stocking.
- The type of hosiery the client normally wears and the mode of suspension.

An important point that must be considered is the dexterity of the client. Although clients may be used to applying thigh length stockings, they may find it impossible to manipulate the stiffer compression stocking. Below knee compression hosiery is usually sufficient for prophylactic use. These stockings are easier to apply correctly, particularly stockings with open toes, and so patients are more encouraged to wear them. Furthermore, stockings or tights may also be worn on top. It is important that clients are warned about constricting bands developing around the leg if used with garters or a knot twisted in the top of the stocking.

If the client's leg circumference below the knee is larger than the calf, they may experience problems keeping below knee stockings up. In these instances, made to measure stockings may be necessary.

## Measuring for elastic hosiery

It is important to measure the client's leg following leg elevation, or early in the day, to minimise the effects of oedema.

For standard sized knee stockings, the following measurements must be taken:

- The ankle circumference of the client at the thinnest point.
- The calf circumference at the widest point.
- The below knee length.
- If the client requires thigh length standard stockings, the measurements are the same as for below knee stockings, but also including the mid-thigh circumference and leg length.

### Made-to-measure hosiery

If standard hosiery does not fit the client, they will need made-to-measure garments. The manufacturers of this hosiery require precise measurements. **Figure 10.4** shows the points at which a leg should be measured for below knee and thigh length made-to-measure stockings. Measurements must be taken systematically from the top to the bottom of the leg. Measurements around the heel should not be forgotten, as this is the widest point of the foot over which the stocking has to pass.

**Length**

10 to 8 and 9 to 8 – draw around the clients foot whilst they are standing on paper. Mark the widest point at toe base (position 9)

11. Point that measurement must be made between the height of each circumference and the floor

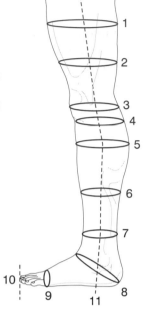

**Circumference**

1. Top of thigh
2. Mid point between 1 and 3
3. Knee at widest point
4. Base of knee i.e. point where below knee stocking ends
5. Widest calf circumference
6. Midpoint between 5 and 7
7. Ankle at narrowest point if it is not possible to identify this point measure 2-4 cm above ankle bone
8. Widest point for stocking to pass
9. Toe base – note any abnormalities

**Figure 10.4**

# Prescribing elastic hosiery

Before the prescription for elastic hosiery can be dispensed, the following details must be provided by the prescriber:

- The quantity – single or pair.
- The article (i.e. style and type including any accessories).
- Compression Class I, II, or III.
- Client measurements if stockings are to be made-to-measure.

## Fitting elastic hosiery

Most clients will need to be shown how to apply compression hosiery. When applying stockings, the garment should be turned inside out as far as the heel. Thumbs should then be inserted into the sides of the stocking and the stocking should be slipped on until the heel is in the correct position. The fabric of the stocking should then be gathered up and gently eased up the ankle and the leg. The thumbs should be kept inside the stocking, and the stocking should be spread as evenly as possible until the knee or thigh is reached. If any tight bands and unevenness are present, these should be gently smoothed away. The stocking should not be folded over, if it is too high, once it has been applied. This would cause a band of constriction. Instead, the stocking must be removed and reapplied.

Open-toed stockings are more easily applied if a silky socklet, supplied by the manufacturer, is first slipped over the forefoot and pulled out when the stocking is in position. Similarly, using the lower part of a nylon stocking over the bare leg may help. Stockings should be removed at night and put on again immediately on rising, before oedema has collected. The exception to this is when stockings are worn for DVT prophylaxis. These stockings should be worn all the time, both during the day and night and may only be removed for up to thirty minutes to allow time for bathing. Some people may feel claustrophobic wearing compression stockings. Therefore, they may need to get used to garments slowly, initially wearing them for one or two hours at a time.

At the first fittings, any modifications need to be noted. If compression therapy is very effective in reducing oedema, then the leg may need to be re-measured after only a few weeks.

Aids are available to help apply elastic hosiery. However, these devices rely on the sight, strength and manual dexterity of the client. Applying elastic hosiery may therefore present problems for those with arthritic hips or hands. A relative or friend may need to be relied upon to help. If two pairs of stockings are worn at the same time, the pressure is cumulative. Therefore, it is sometimes advisable to recommend that clients wear two pairs of Class 1 stocking as opposed to a Class III stocking. They are easier to apply and equally as effective (Fentem, 1986).

### Washing elastic hosiery

All articles provide clear washing instructions, which conform to hand-washing at 40°C. It is important that these instructions are followed if hosiery is to maintain its correct compression. Frequent daily washing improves performance by restoring shape and removing damaging skin oils. With good care, stockings should give adequate pressure for three or four months before needing to be replaced.

## CONTRAINDICATIONS

Compression therapy should never be applied in clients with severe arteriosclerosis or any other ischaemic vascular disease. Also, stocking should not be worn if there are any local conditions affecting the leg (e.g. skin lesions, gangrenous conditions, or recent vein ligation), as they may compromise the circulation.

The fibres used to make modern stockings rarely cause allergies. If a client has a very sensitive skin a patch test should be performed. The manufacturer can be contacted in order to obtain a sample of stocking to perform the test.

# References

Fentem, P.H. (1986). Elastic hosiery. *Pharmacy Update* 5: 200–205.

Drug Tarriff (1998). National Health Service England and Wales. London: The Stationery Office.

# 11

# FOLIC ACID

Nurse prescribers can play an important role in the health care of women of a reproductive age. They can promote the chances of a positive pregnancy outcome by ensuring women are aware of the importance of folic acid supplementation and an adequate dietary intake of folic acid, and should prescribe folic acid to women where appropriate. This chapter considers the role of folic acid in preventing neural tube defects (NTDs) and current recommendations for folic acid intake during pregnancy.

## FORMATION OF THE NEURAL TUBE

During the third week of development following fertilisation of an ovum, the process of gastrulation occurs. This is the formation of the three primary germ layers (ectoderm, mesoderm and endoderm) in the developing embryo. Gastrulation provides the basic framework for organogenesis or the formation of organs and organ systems in the embryo. The central nervous system (CNS) which consists of the brain and spinal cord, develops from the ectoderm. The differentiation of the ectoderm into the CNS is refered to as neurulation.

The ectoderm thickens to form the neural plate. The plate then begins to fold inwards and forms a longitudinal groove called the neural groove. The raised edges of the neural plate are called neural folds. Continuing development of the neural folds results in the folds meeting to form a tube called the neural tube (**Figure 11.1**). The neural tube then detaches from the surface ectoderm to lie beneath it. The tube undergoes elongation and changes in its shape. The anterior end of the neural tube develops into the brain and

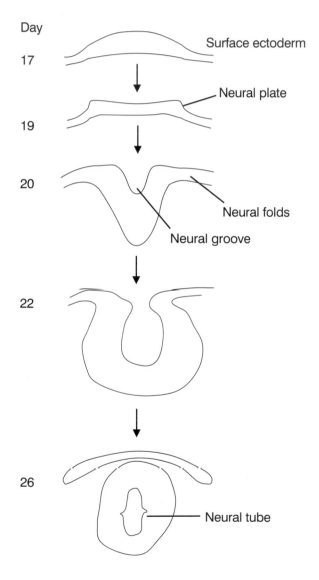

**Figure 11.1** – Development of the neural tube

the posterior section becomes the spinal cord. The cavity of the neural tube becomes the central canal of the spinal cord and expands at the head to become the ventricles of the brain.

## NEURAL TUBE DEFECTS

Failure of the neural tube to close correctly, leads to a group of conditions called neural tube defects. These defects include anencephaly, encephalocele and spina bifida. In anencephaly, the soft bony component of the skull and part of the brain are missing. Infants with anencephaly are usually stillborn or die shortly after birth. Encephalocele is herniation of the brain and meninges through a defect in the skull. The size, location and involvement of the encephalocele will assist in determining the overall effect on the infant's physical and intellectual development. Spina bifida results from incomplete closure of the neural tube with an associated malformation of the vertebral column. The spinal cord and meninges may or may not protrude.

NTDs are among the most common, severe, congenital malformations and the United Kingdom has one of the highest rates of NTDs in the world (Medical Research Council, 1991). It is quite likely that most cases of NTD occur because of a combination of unknown genetic and environmental factors, both of which must be triggered for the NTD to occur (Seller, 1987).

## FOLIC ACID

Folic acid (folate) is a water-soluble vitamin involved in a variety of metabolic reactions. It acts as a carrier of methyl groups and will carry one-carbon units from one molecule to another. The metabolism of folic acid is closely linked to that of vitamin $B_{12}$ and vitamin $B_{12}$ deficiency will result in secondary folic acid deficiency (Bender, 1993). Folate deficiency affects rapidly dividing cells, particularly those of the bone marrow, intestinal mucosa and hair follicles. Clinically, folic acid deficiency leads to a megaloblastic anaemia where large, immature red blood cells are released from the bone marrow.

### Role of folic acid in prevention of NTDs

It has been suspected for some time that diet, and specifically folic acid, may have a role in the development of NTDs. Studies by Laurence *et al* (1981) and Smithells *et al* (1983) indicated that pre-conception folic acid or other vitamin supplementation might reduce the incidence of a recurrence of NTD in women who already have had one child with NTD. Results of work by the Medical Research Council (1991) confirmed a link between folic acid and the development of NTDs. Providing pre-conception folic acid supplementation to women who had previously given birth to an affected infant, reduced the risk of a further such affected pregnancy by 72%.

Evidence for the role of folic acid in preventing occurences of NTD in women expecting their first child was not clear. However, Czeizel and Dudas (1992) performed a randomised, controlled trial which concluded that a pre-conceptional multivitamin supplementation (containing folic acid) decreased the incidence of a first occurrence of NTD. In 1992, an Expert Advisory Group from the Department of Health published recommendations regarding folic acid supplementation and dietary folic acid, for all women planning a pregnancy.

The requirement for extra folate in relation to NTDs may be because of an interaction between a folic acid dependency and a dietary deficiency (Czeizel, 1995). Localised folic acid deficiency in the embryo may lead to impaired cell division at the time of neural tube closure. However, the actual mechanism by which folic acid assists in prevention of, but does not eliminate the risk of NTDs still remains to be elucidated (Sadler, 1995).

### Recommended requirements for folic acid during pregnancy

The reference nutrient intake (RNI) for folic acid in non-pregnant women is currently 200 μg per day.

All women who are planning a pregnancy should take a daily supplement of 400 μg folic acid from around the time of conception and for the first three months of pregnancy. In addition, they should try to eat 300 μg of folic acid daily. Examples of good dietary sources of folic acid can be seen in **Table 11.1**. Care should be taken not to over cook vegetables as this reduces their folic acid content.

Women who have unplanned pregnancies should be told to take 400 μg as soon as they realise they are pregnant, and until the twelfth week of pregnancy. Dietary intake of folic acid should also be increased to 300 μg.

Women who have had a previous pregnancy resulting in an infant with a NTD, will require a higher dose of folic acid (5 mg). This is only available on prescription from a physician. These women should also try to consume a diet with adequate folic acid.

**Table 11.1** – *Dietary Sources of Folate*

| Food Source | μg folic acid per average serving |
|---|---|
| Bran flakes | 113 |
| Cornflakes | 88 |
| Rice Krispies | 88 |
| All Bran | 86 |
| | |
| Brussel sprouts | 127 |
| Spinach | 117 |
| Broccoli | 61 |
| Green beans | 59 |
| Cauliflower | 51 |
| Potatoes | 45 |
| Orange juice | 40 |
| | |
| Bread (white, 2 slices) | 70 |
| Bread (granary, 2 slices) | 68 |
| Bread (wholemeal 2 slices) | 29 |
| | |
| Black-eye beans | 220 |
| Soya beans | 59 |
| Chick peas | 59 |
| Red kidney beans | 44 |
| | |
| Cottage cheese | 40 |
| Yoghurt (low fat, fruit) | 24 |
| Milk (semi-skimmed, pint) | 35 |
| | |
| Marmite | 50 |
| Bovril | 50 |

# References

Bender D.A. (1993) – *Introduction to Nutrition and Metabolism.* London: UCL Press.

Czeizel A.E. (1995) – Folic acid in the prevention of neural tube defects. *Journal of Pediatric Gastroenterology and Nutrition* 20: 4–16.

Czeizel A.E. and Dudas I. (1992) – Prevention of the first occurrence of neural tube defects by periconceptional vitamin supplementation. *New England Journal of Medicine* 327 (26): 1832–1835.

Department of Health Expert Advisory Group (1992) – *Folic acid and the prevention of neural tube defects.* London: Department of Health.

Laurence K.M., James N., Miller M.H., Tennant G.B. and Cambell H. (1981) – Double-blind randomised controlled trial of folate treatment before conception to prevent recurrence of neural tube defects. *British Medical Journal* 282: 1509–1511.

Medical Research Council Vitamin Study Research Group (1991) – Prevention of neural tube defects: Results of the Medical Research Council Vitamin Study. *The Lancet* 338: 131–137.

Sadler M.J. (1995) – Folic acid and NTDs – moving forwards. *BNF Nutrition Bulletin* 20: 93–95.

Seller M.J. (1987) – Nutritionally induced congenital defects. *Procedings of Nutrition Society* 46 (2): 227–235.

Smithells R.W., Seller M.J., Harris R., Fielding D.W., Schorah C.J., Nevin N.C., Sheppard S., Read A.P., Walker S. and Wild J. (1983) – Further experience of vitamin supplementation for prevention of neural tube defect recurrences. *The Lancet* 1: 1027–1031.

# Appendix 1

## GLOSSARY OF TERMS

**Action potential:** The distinctive change in voltage between the inside and outside of neurones and muscle cells, initiated by a change in the membrane permeability to sodium ions.

**Active transport:** The input of energy to excrete or absorb solutes across a cell membrane.

**Adverse reaction:** Unfavourable response.

**Aerosol:** A suspension of very small droplets of a liquid, or particles of a solid, in air.

**Agonist:** Drugs that are similar in structure to natural neurotransmitters which bind to a receptor and activate it.

**Analgesic:** A drug that relieves pain.

**Antacid:** Alkaline preparation that counteracts the strong acid environment in the stomach.

**Antagonist:** A substance similar in structure to a natural neurotransmitter, which bind to a receptor without activating it. They consequently block the transmission of nerve impulses.

**Arteriosclerosis:** A thickening and toughening of arterial walls.

**Biofilm:** A collection of micro-organisms and their products on a solid surface.

**Biotransformation:** The process of modifying or altering the chemical composition of a drug.

**Cardiac output:** The quantity of blood ejected by the left ventricle each minute; approximately 5 litres.

**Cerebrospinal fluid:** The fluid which bathes the internal and external surfaces of the central nervous system.

**Contraindication:** Anything which makes a proposed form of medical intervention undesirable or dangerous.

**Deep fascia:** Connective tissue fibres that form sheets beneath the skin to stabilise, attach, enclose and separate muscles and other internal organs.

**Diffusion:** The passive movement of molecules from an area of relatively high concentration to an area of relatively low concentration.

**Diuretic:** A substance which increases the urine flow rate.

**Emulsions:** A fluid formed by the suspension of one liquid in another.

**Enteric coating:** A special coating applied to tablets or capsules, which prevents release and absorption of their content until they reach the intestine.

**Enterohepatic circulation:** Bile salt excretion by the liver, followed by absorption of bile salts by the intestinal cells for return to the liver by the hepatic portal vein.

**Enzyme:** A protein that accelerates a specific biochemical reaction.

**Excoriation:** A scratching or abrasion injury to the surface of the body.

**Exudate:** The fluid from blood vessels that usually escapes in the course of inflammation.

**Fermentation:** The breakdown of complex molecules in organic compounds, caused by bacteria.

**First pass effect:** The removal of a drug by the liver, before it is available for use.

**Granulation:** The new tissue formed in repair of wounds of soft tissue.

**Haemolysis:** The breakdown of red blood cells.

**Half-life:** The time taken for the concentration of a drug in the blood to fall by half (50%) its original value.

**Hydrophilic:** Associating freely with water and readily entering into solution.

**Hyperkeratosis:** Thickening of the outer layer of the skin so as to produce a horny layer.

**Hypersensitivity:** An overreaction to an allergen resulting in inflammation and tissue damage.

**Insecticide:** Any substance used to kill insects.

**Ion channels:** The channels through which water soluble molecules and ions can pass through cell membranes.

**Ischaemia:** Inadequate blood supply to a structure of the body.

**Laxatives:** Drugs used to relieve constipation

**Maceration:** To soften and break down

**Melaena:** Stools containing blood.

**Metabolism:** The sum of all of the biochemical processes going on within the body at a given time.

**Mucous membranes:** The inner lining of many of the cavities and hollow internal organs of the body.

**Necrotic tissue:** Dead tissue.

**Neuromuscular junction:** The junction between a nerve terminal and a skeletal muscle fibre.

**Neurotransmitter:** A chemical released by a neurone which affect the activity of another neurone.

**Oedema:** Excessive accumulation of fluid, mainly water, in the body.

**Opportunistic infection:** Infection by organisms that are normally effectively repelled by the body's defence mechanisms, but which are able to establish themselves because these mechanisms are temporarily or permanently defective.

**Osmosis:** The passage of water across a semi-permeable membrane from one solution towards another solution that contains a higher solute concentration.

**Parasite:** Organisms living on or in the body of another living organism.

**Parenteral administration:** The administration of drugs by a route other than the alimentary canal.

**Peristalsis:** Smooth muscle contractions that occur in waves and propel material along such structures as the ureters or digestive tract.

**pH:** The concentration of hydrogen ions in a fluid expressed in moles per litre.

**Pharmacodynamics:** The effects of a drug on the body and the mode of drug action.

**Pharmacokinetics:** The movement of drugs within the body and the way in which the body affects drugs with time.

**Platelets:** Cellular fragments whose main function is sealing off leaks in blood vessels.

**Primary intention healing:** Wounds which can be closed by suturing and require only the formation of a small quantity of new tissue. This process is accomplished within several days.

**Pruritus:** Itching.

**Pulmonary circulation:** The blood circulation through the lungs.

**Pyrexia:** A fever.

**Receptor:** A molecule found on the surface of a cell or located within the cytoplasm. This will bind with specific molecules producing some effect within the cell.

**Reference nutrient intake (RNI):** An intake of a nutrient two standard deviations above the observed mean requirement, and hence greater then the requirements of 97.5% of the population.

**Resistance:** The ability to ward off disease.

**Secondary intention healing:** Wounds in which there is tissue loss, and healing involves the formation of new tissue. This process can take weeks or months.

**Side effects:** The undesirable or dangerous effects produced by a form of medical intervention.

**Sinus:** A cavity in a tissue.

**Slough:** Dead tissue, which is being or has been cast off or separated from its original site.

**Sphincter:** A ring of muscle, which contracts to close the exit or entrance of an internal passage.

**Sterile:** Free from living micro-organisms.

**Sublingual:** Under the tongue.

**Suppositories:** Medication administered via the rectal route.

**Symbiosis:** The living together of two kinds of organisms to their mutual advantage.

**Systemic circulation:** The circulatory system other than those of the pulmonary circulation.

**Teratogen:** Any agent that will cause physical defects in a developing embryo.

**Therapeutic effect:** The extent to which an intervention aids the well being of an individual.

**Therapeutic index:** The ratio of a drug's toxic dose to its minimally effective dose.

**Topical (medication):** Applied to the body surface.

**Toxic effects:** Poisonous effects.

**Transdermal:** Through the skin.

**Transit time:** The time taken for stools to travel through the colon.

**Vasoconstriction:** The contraction of smooth muscle causing a reduction in the diameter of arterioles.

# Appendix 2

## NURSE PRESCRIBERS' LIST

List of preparations approved by the Secretary of State which may be prescribed on forms FP10CN and FP10PN (forms GP10(CN) and GP10(PN) in Scotland, form HS21(N) in Northern Ireland) by Nurses for National Health Service Patients

### Medicinal Preparations

Almond Oil Ear Drops, NPF
Arachis Oil Enema, NPF
Aspirin Tablets, Dispersible, 300mg, BP
Bisacodyl Suppositories, BP (includes 5-mg and 10-mg strengths)
Bisacodyl Tablets, BP
Cadexomer – Iodine Ointment, NPF
Cadexomer – Iodine Paste, NPF
Cadexomer – Iodine Powder, NPF
Calamine Cream, Aqueous, BP
Calamine Lotion, BP
Calamine Lotion, Oily, BP 1980
Catheter Maintenance Solution, Chlorhexidine, NPF
Catheter Maintenance Solution, Mandelic Acid, NPF
Catheter Maintenance Solution, Sodium Chloride, NPF

Catheter Maintenance Solution, 'Solution G', NPF
Catheter Maintenance Solution, 'Solution R', NPF
Clotrimazole Cream 1%, BP
Co-danthramer Capsules, NPF
Co-danthramer Capsules, Strong, NPF
Co-danthramer Oral Suspension, NPF
Co-danthramer Oral Suspension, Strong, NPF
Co-danthrusate Capsules, BP
Co-danthrusate Oral Suspension, NPF
Dextranomer Beads, NPF
Dextranomer Paste, NPF
Dimethicone barrier creams containing at least 10%
Docusate Capsules, NPF
Docusate Enema, NPF
Docusate Enema, Compound, NPF
Docusate Oral Solution, NPF
Docusate Oral Solution, Paediatric, NPF
Econazole Cream 1%, BP
Emollients as listed below:
    Alcoderm® Cream
    Alcoderm® Lotion
    Aqueous Cream, BP
    Dermamist®
    Diprobase® Cream
    Diprobase® Ointment
    E45® Cream
    Emulsifying Ointment, BP
    Epaderm®
    Humiderm® Cream
    Hydromol ® Cream
    Hydrous Ointment, BP
    Keri® Therapeutic Lotion
    LactiCare® Lotion
    Lipobase®
    Neutrogena® Dermatological Cream
    Oilatum® Cream
    Ultrabase®
    †Unguentum Merck®
Emollient Bath Additives as listed below:
    Alpha Keri® Bath Oil
    †Balneum®
    Diprobath®
    Emmolate® Bath Oil
    Hydromol® Emollient

Oilatum ® Emollient
Oilatum® Gel
Folic Acid Tablets 400 micrograms, BP
Glycerol Suppositories, BP
Ispaghula Husk Granules, NPF
Ispaghula Husk Granules, Effervescent, NPF
Ispaghula Husk Powder, NPF
Lactitol Powder, NPF
Lactulose Powder, NPF
Lactulose Solution, BP
Lignocaine Gel, BP
Lignocaine Ointment, NPF
Lignocaine and Chlorhexidine Gel, BP
Magnesium Hydroxide Mixture, BP
Magnesium Sulphate Paste, BP
Malathoin alcoholic lotions containing at least 0.5%
Malathion aqueous lotions containing at least 0.5%
Mebendazole Oral Suspension, NPF
Mebendazole Tablets, NPF
Miconazole Cream 2%, BP
Miconazole Oral Gel, NPF
Nystatin Oral Suspension, BP
Nystatin Pastilles, NPF
Olive Oil Ear Drops, NPF
Paracetamol Oral Suspension, BP (includes 120 mg/5mL and 250 mg/5mL
     strengths-both of which are available as sugar-free formulations)
Paracetamol Tablets, BP
Paracetamol Tablets, Soluble, BP
Permethrin Cream, NPF
Permethrin Cream Rinse, NPF
Phenothrin Alcoholic Lotion, NPF
Phosphates Enema, BP
Piperazine Citrate Elixir, BP
Piperazine and Senna Powder, NPF
Povidone-Iodine Solution, BP
Senna Granules, Standardised, BP
Senna Oral Solution, NPF
Senna Tablets, BP
Senna and Ispaghula Granules, NPF
Sodium Chloride Solution, Sterile,BP
Sodium Citrate Compound Enema, NPF
Sodium Picosulphate Elixir, NPF
Sterculia Granules, NPF
Sterculia and Frangula Granules, NPF

Streptokinase and Streptodornase Topical Powder, NPF
Thymol Glycerin, Compound, BP 1988
Titanium Ointment, NPF
Zinc and Castor Oil Ointment, BP
Zinc Oxide and Dimethicone Spray, NPF
Zinc Oxide Impregnated Medicated Stocking, NPF

## Appliances and Reagents (including Wound Management Products)

In the Drug Tariff appliances and Reagents which may not be prescribed by
Nurses are annotated N (Nx in the Scottish Drug Tariff and NHS in the Northern
Ireland Drug Tariff)

## Chemical Reagents

The following as listed in Part IXR of the Drug Tariff (Part 9 of the Scottish
Drug Tariff, Part II of the Northern Ireland Drug Tariff):
    Detection Tablets for Glycosuria
    Detection Tablets for Ketonuria
    Detection Strips for Glycosuria
    Detection Strips for Ketonuria
    Detection Strips for Proteinuria
    Detection Strips for Blood Glucose
    Also in BNF section 6.1.6 Items not in the Drug Tariff (and thus not
    prescribable) are described as NHS in the BNF. Although glucose for glucose
    tolerance test is in section 6.1.6 it is not on the Nurse Prescribers' List

Fertility (Ovulation) Thermometer as listed under Contraceptive Devices in Part
I XA of the Drug Tariff (Part 3 of the Scottish Drug Tariff, Part III of the
Northern Ireland Drug Tariff)
Corresponds to Fertility Thermometer in BNF section 7.3.4
Film Gloves, Disposable, EMA as listed under Protectives in Part IXA of the
Drug Tariff (Part 2 of the Scottish Drug Tariff, Part III of the Northern Ireland
Drug Tariff)
Elastic Hosiery including accessories as listed in Part IXA of the Drug Tariff
(Part 4 of the Scottish Drug Tariff, Part III of the Northern Ireland Drug Tariff)
Also in BNF Appendix 9

## Hypodermic Equipment

The following as listed in Part IXA of the Drug Tariff (Part 3 of the Scottish
Drug Tariff, Part III of the Northern Ireland Drug Tariff):
    Hypodermic Syringes-U100 Insulin
    Hypodermic Syringe-Single Use of Single-patient Use, U100 Insulin with
    needle
    Hypodermic Needles-Sterile, Single-use

Lancets-Sterile, Single-use
Needle Clipping Device
Also in BNF section 6.1.1.3. Items not in the Drug Tariff (and thus not
    prescribable) are described as NHS in the BNF
Incontinence Appliances as listed in Part IXB of the Drug Tariff (Part 5 of the
    Scottish Drug Tariff, Part III of the Northern Ireland Drug Tariff)
    Also in BNF appendix 8: Incontinence Appliances
Irrigation Fluids as listed in Part IXA of the Drug Tariff (Part 2 of the Scottish
    Drug Tariff, Part III of the Northern Ireland Drug Tariff)
Pessaries, Ring as listed in Part IXA of the Drug Tariff (Part 3 of the Scottish
    Drug Tariff, Part III of the Northern Ireland Drug Tariff)
Stoma Appliances and Associated Products as listed in Part IXC of the Drug
    Tariff (Part 6 of the Scottish Drug Tariff, Part III of the Northern Ireland
    drug Tariff)
Also in BNF Appendix 8: Soma Appliances
Urethral Catheters as listed under Catheters in Part IXA of the Drug Tariff (Part
    3 of the Scottish Drug Tariff, Part III of the Northern Ireland Drug Tariff
Also in BNF appendix 8: Urethral Catheters
Urine Sugar Analysis Equipment as listed in Part IXA of the Drug Tariff (Parts 3
    and 9 of the Scottish Drug Tariff, Part III of the Northern Ireland Drug
    Tariff)
Also in BNF section 6.1.6

## *Wound Management and Related Products*

(Including bandages, dressings, gauzes, lint, stockinette, etc)
The following as listed in Part IXA of the Drug Tariff (Part 2 of the Scottish
Drug Tariff, Part III of the Northern Ireland Drug Tariff):

Absorbent Cottons
Absorbent Cotton Gauzes
Absorbent Cotton and Viscose Ribbon Gauze, BP 1988
Absorbent Lint, BPC
Absorbent Perforated Plastic Film Faced Dressing
Arm Slings
Cellulose Wadding, BP 1988
Cotton Conforming Bandage, BP 1988
Cotton Crêpe Bandage, BP 1988
Cotton Polyamide and Elastane Bandage
Crépe Bandage, BP 1988
Elastic Adhesive Bandage, BP 1988
Elastic Web Bandages
Elastomer and Viscose Bandage, Knitted
Gauze and Cotton Tissues
Heavy Cotton and Rubber Elastic Bandage, BP

High Compression Bandages (Extensible)
Knitted Polyamide and Cellulose Contour Bandage, BP 1988
Knitted Viscose Primary Dressing, BP, Type 1
Multiple Pack Dressing No.1
Multiple Pack Dressing No.2
Open-wove Bandage, BP 1988, Type 1
Paraffin Gauze Dressing, BP
Polyamide and Cellulose Contour Bandage, BP 1988
Povidone-Iodine Fabric Dressing, Sterile
Skin Closure Strips, Sterile
Sterile Dressing Packs
Stockinettes
Surgical Adhesive Tapes
Suspensory Bandages, Cotton
Swabs
Triangular Calico Bandage, BP 1980
Vapour-permeable Adhesive Film Dressing, BP
Vapour-permeable Waterproof Plastic Wound Dressing, BP, Sterile
Wound Management Dressings (including alignate, hydrocolloid, hydrogel and foam)
Zinc Paste Bandages (including both plain and with additional ingredient)

Also in BNF Appendix 9. Items are not in the Drug Tariff (and thus not prescribable) are described as NHS in the BNF. Although Chlorhexidine Gauze Dressing BP, Framycetin Gauze Dressing BP, and Sodium Fusidate Gauze Dressing BP, are in Appendix 9 they are not on the Nurse Prescribers'List.

1.  Except pack sizes that are not to be prescribed under the NHS (see Part XV111A of the Drug Tariff Part XI of the Northern Ireland Drug Tariff)

# INDEX